# CNA Study Guide 2020-2021

*Exam Prep with 240 Test Questions and Answers for the Certified Nursing Assistant Exam (Including Detailed Answer Explanations for 4 Practice Tests)*

Published by Newstone TestPrep

ISBN 978-1-989726-00-6 (Paperback)

# Table of Contents

# Chapter 1: CNA at a Glance

A Certified Nursing Assistant (CNA) is a professional who works under the supervision of a qualified nurse. CNAs are in direct contact with patients and provide care such as helping individuals to bathe, taking their vital signs and helping them move around.

They also serve meals and often help patients eat, reposition them when they are bedridden, provide clean bedpans and empty used ones, answer calls, check for bruises, examine urine for signs of blood, sanitize common areas, change bed linen and restock rooms with required provisions.

## Who is Qualified to Take the CNA Exam?

CNAs, though certified as nursing assistants, are not licensed to practice as health care workers. Their role is to assist qualified nurses such as registered nurses, licensed practical nurses or licensed vocational nurses in providing care. For example, CNAs can change bedding but cannot administer medication.

The qualifications required in order to take the CNA exam vary from state to state, but the one common requirement is a high school diploma. After that, potential candidates attend a six- to eight-week training program designed to prepare them for their role in the health care field. Program graduates can then register for the CNA exam. Those who pass the exam receive certification and from then on are referred to as CNAs. This certification helps CNAs secure employment in hospitals, nursing homes, long-term care facilities, institutions offering home-based care and other places.

## Format of the CNA Exam & Time Allowed

The CNA exam is made up of a writing section and a practical skills section.

### The Written Part of the CNA Exam

The written part of the CNA exam is meant to test a candidate's understanding of general nursing concepts. The section has 60 questions, and candidates have one and a half hours to complete them.

### The CNA Exam Practical Skills Part

This part of the CNA exam takes 30 minutes. During that time you are expected to demonstrate competence in approximately five clinical skills. During the test, a proctor will monitor the room to ensure clinical skills are being executed appropriately. Precision is key to this portion of the exam.

Don't panic if you realize you've made a mistake during a procedure. Instead, inform the proctor that you have made a mistake and want to correct it. He or she will allow you to do so in order to ensure you demonstrate that you really understand how to execute the relevant clinical skill.

### Timing and Passing Score

It's important to note that the times given for each section of the CNA exam in this chapter are fairly standard, but those times can occasionally vary from state to state.

In terms of a passing score, 70 percent is the required minimum, but again, this can vary by state.

## The Tasks a CNA Carries Out on a Daily Basis

Although CNAs are not licensed to perform tasks of a medical nature, they have many daily responsibilities that involve assisting patients with tasks that are generally easy for healthy people but difficult when a person is ailing, weak or elderly. A good example of such tasks is bathing.

Other tasks CNAs are responsible for include helping patients shave, brush their teeth, eat, dress and ambulate. CNAs are expected to know how to empty a used catheter and a colostomy bag. They should also have the necessary skills for application and removal of patients' splints and braces. Since they are also charged with taking patients' vital signs, CNAs are expected to know how to use blood pressure cuffs, stethoscopes and electronic thermometers.

In addition to being competent and certified, CNAs must also be compassionate and patient. They are expected to have great communication skills both in order to assist their patients and also to clearly convey patients' challenges to supervisors as needed.

In some cases, CNAs are required to use software for the purposes of billing patients, managing patients' individual information and charting medical records. After in-house training, some CNAs are given additional responsibilities that are intended as stepping stones to further formal training and career advancement. It's important that CNAs always operate within the bounds of the law, state policy and facility regulations.

### Maintaining Safety

Keeping patients safe constitutes a big part of a CNA's job. It's imperative that CNAs protect not only their patients but also themselves from injury or infection. It's also important that they have the relevant skills to feed patients who have difficulties in swallowing, to prevent choking or aspiration. CNAs are often called upon to move patients from their respective beds to their wheelchairs and vice-versa. Therefore they should be skilled in assisting patients with moving around safely. Other clients may not be so disabled but might still be too weak to walk on their own, and therefore it is the duty of a CNA to help such individuals leave bed and sit on a chair, leave the chair and go enjoy some sunshine, etc.

CNAs working in long-term health care facilities, residential homes and other such places are also required to recognize patient abuse and to immediately report such cases to their supervisors.

# Expected Level of Medical Knowledge

CNAs are not expected to be vastly knowledgeable in medical matters, but they are expected to understand basic human anatomy and physiology. They are also required to have basic knowledge of the major body systems and the diseases likely to affect each of them.

For example, they are expected to be able to identify potential instances of melanoma (skin cancer) and to recognize signs of possible illness such as pallor and weight loss. While CNAs can't treat such conditions, their ability to refer patients to qualified medical professionals for prompt care is invaluable.

### Expected Knowledge of Infections

It's important that CNAs be knowledgeable about infectious diseases not only so that they can help prevent infected patients from infecting others, but also in order to protect themselves in the course of duty. CNAs are expected to be familiar with basic infection prevention techniques, which include thorough and frequent handwashing, disposing of soiled items appropriately and when and how to make use of protective gear such as masks, gowns and gloves. In the same context of infection control, CNAs are expected to be able to read signs of infection in patients which include abnormally elevated body temperature, diarrhea and an unresolving cough.

# CNAs' Role in Emergencies

CNAs should be skilled in performing cardio-pulmonary resuscitation (CPR) in the event that a patient suffers a heart attack or has breathing difficulties.

Additionally, CNAs should know how to stop bleeding and be familiar with what to do if an unconscious patient starts to vomit. They should also know how to call for emergency help from a hospital, nursing facility or relevant health care institution.

# Chapter 2: Becoming a CNA

Compared to other health care careers, becoming a CNA is relatively easy. For starters, the fact that you don't need a college degree to take the CNA exam is an advantage to many.

## What You Need to Qualify for the CNA Exam

As we noted earlier, all you need in order to qualify to take the CNA exam is a high school diploma. Those who don't have a high school diploma can present proof of taking the GED test or an equivalent exam. You may be required to provide high school transcripts.

In addition to having a high school diploma or its equivalent, you may be required to take an entrance exam at the college you're trying to enroll in for your CNA program. While not all schools offering CNA training have such a requirement, it's good to be aware of it. Additionally, some schools also do a background check for any kind of criminal history.

## CNA Preparatory Course Accreditation

State accreditation for a CNA preparatory program indicates that the program is highly regarded and has met the educational standards for nursing recognized at a national level. The longer the program has been accredited, the more confident you can be that it's a high quality course. Many accredited institutions that offer CNA programs also have higher-level nursing courses, and this means you should be able to easily enroll for later training if that's of interest to you.

One more advantage of enrolling in an accredited program is that you stand a better chance of receiving financial assistance. State funds can't be used to sponsor students in programs that the state has not approved.

### *Exam Preparation*

When preparing for the CNA exam, a lot of practice is required in tackling the kinds of questions presented on the test, and that's where books like this one come in handy. After all, the preparatory programs offered in various schools are quite short, yet there is a broad spectrum of topics to be covered. While a good program will teach you the basics required to be a CNA, you may still wish to do more practice answering questions on geriatrics, physiology and other such topics. Not only will that help with your exam preparation, but it can only help you when you take a position as a certified CNA.

# What Happens After the CNA Exam?

Once you have passed the CNA exam, you are recognized as a Certified Nursing Assistant, and your name is included in the registry of the state where you took the test.

Certification is important as it provides assurance to potential employers that you have the required level of knowledge and skills to take care of patients. For example, passing the exam tells employers that you're able to take vital signs, can effectively handle an emergency and can fulfill the health care responsibilities CNAs are expected to shoulder.

As a CNA there are many job opportunities available, and they only get better if you opt to specialize in a particular discipline. For example, when you are already practicing as a CNA, you can choose to study and be certified in geriatrics. Such credentials are an advantage when it comes to finding better-paying jobs.

## CNA Recertification

After working as a CNA for two years, you need to be recertified by the relevant state body. To qualify for such recertification, you have to provide proof that you've completed a minimum of 48 hours of continuing education.

Some states require a minimum of 12 hours of continuing education hours for each year. It is presumed that in those hours you will receive training in areas of health care importance such as domestic violence, first aid and patients' rights, as well as in keeping medical records. Many employers pay for CNAs' required continuing education.

## Length of a CNA Course

In general, CNA programs last from four to 12 weeks. CNA programs that have been approved by the state offer at least 75 hours of instruction in a classroom in addition to the mandatory clinical training. Some colleges split the program such that students spend four weeks receiving instruction in class and then undergo practical training within a clinical setting for two weeks.

## Jobs Available for CNAs

There are many job opportunities for CNAs in the United States, and according to recent statistics, the trend is likely to continue up to 2026. According to America's Bureau of Labor Statistics, employment for CNAs is bound to keep rising by more than 10 percent owing to factors like an aging population, the growing popularity of nursing homes and a rise in a population suffering from chronic illnesses.

Some sectors likely to continue requiring high numbers of CNAs are home-based and community-based health care providers.

### *Home-based Health Care Environment*

Some CNAs opt to work in home-based health care, where CNAs take care of individual patients rather than caring for multiple individuals.

When working in a home-based environment, you can anticipate a less hectic schedule, but your pay is also likely to be a bit lower than for CNAs working in busier environments. It's more challenging to juggle the demands of several patients, and so the difference in pay compensates for that.

### *The Hospital Environment*

Many CNA candidates hope to work in hospitals because they often offer good benefits and the pay is comparatively higher than elsewhere. In addition, the hospital environment allows CNAs to work alongside (and learn from) a range of medical personnel. Hospitals also provide opportunities for working in a variety of departments that can broaden a CNA's skill set.

One downside to working in a large institution such as a hospital is that you may not have a chance to form long-term relationships with the patients you care for. Hospital patients are brought in with the aim of receiving treatment and being discharged rather quickly. Conversely, clients often spend years in nursing homes and form rich relationships with the CNAs who take care of them.

## Opportunities CNAs Have for Advancement

CNAs can always return to college for further training to become registered or licensed nurses. Here are some of the qualifications CNAs can acquire throughout the course of their career.

### *Licensed Practical Nurse (LPN)*

Licensed Practical Nurses are one level higher than CNAs. Therefore, they can perform certain tasks that CNAs cannot and earn slightly higher salaries that are commensurate with that skill level.

### *Occupational Therapy Assistant (OTA)*

Just like CNAs work under qualified nurses, Occupational Therapy Assistants (OTAs) work under occupational therapists (OTs). OTAs' role is to assist patients undergoing occupational therapy to regain or improve daily life skills.

### *Personal Care Aides*

Personal Care Aides not only assist their clients to perform important daily tasks, but they also serve as clients' close companions. This means their presence is required even when those clients have other health care workers who provide them with basic health care within the home environment.

## CNAs' Salaries

Though a new CNA's salary isn't exactly impressive, the salary should not be a deterrent from pursuing the career path because of how much room there is for growth. For many people holding well-paying jobs in the medical profession, becoming a CNA was what first opened doors for them.

### *Average Salary per Year*

Going by the figures from the US Bureau of Labor Statistics (BLS), a CNA's annual salary averages $26,590, although actual salaries for individuals vary depending on each person's specialization in a given field, workstation, length of experience and a range of other factors.

Per the BLS, 10 percent of all CNAs earn salaries of $36,170 or more annually. The beauty of becoming a CNA is that once you have been certified, you can only go higher in the medical profession and can easily progress to becoming a licensed practical nurse, a licensed vocational nurse or even a registered nurse.

# Chapter 3: The 20-plus Skills Tested in the CNA Exam

Before you think of becoming a CNA, you must be certain you are passionate about helping others. You must be the kind of person who isn't likely to tire of caring for patients at a personal level even when their cases are serious or sensitive. If that describes you, then taking a CNA course and passing the certification exam is all that stands between you and your career dream.

Although certification for CNAs varies somewhat in different states, there are specific skills that almost every state tests. These include hygiene, infection control, nutrition, suitable workplace behavior and restorative services. Candidates are also tested on how best to handle patients' mental, spiritual and cultural needs. Topics pertaining to communication between CNAs and patients, patients' rights and ethical workplace behavior are all common sources of CNA exam questions.

## Skills Tested in Section One: the Written CNA Exam

Specific skills tested in the written section of the CNA exam include:

- anatomy and physiology
- patient nutrition
- patient safety
- infection control
- measuring vital signs
- the aging process
- mental health
- patients' personal care
- patients' rights
- matters pertaining to communication
- issues of an ethical or legal nature
- matters related to patients' daily activities
- mechanics of the body in general
- handling of patients' needs of a cultural or spiritual nature.

You can also anticipate questions pertaining to range of motion, CNAs' role and duties in relation to patients, collection of data and knowledge of medical terminology.

## Skills Tested in Section Two: the Practical CNA Exam

The practical part of the CNA exam challenges you to accurately and efficiently demonstrate various clinical skills.

Skills candidates may be tested on include:

- taking a patient's blood pressure and recording the results
- feeding patients
- bathing or dressing patients
- helping a patient to use a bedpan
- assisting a patient with exercises pertaining to range of motion
- providing a patient with catheter care.

During this practical part of the exam, candidates are expected to also demonstrate proper handwashing techniques and also to show that they understand the need to wash hands before attending to a patient and immediately after. Candidates will also be tested on their skills in communicating and interacting with patients.

## What Else to Expect in the Clinical Skills Test

As you go through your CNA preparatory course, you will learn over 20 skills. Nevertheless, as you can imagine, the time allocated for the CNA questions is not sufficient for you to demonstrate how good you are at every single required skill. For that reason, once you have registered for the exam, a computer program will determine the particular skills you will be tested on. There may up to be five of these.

Given that CNA tasks can be carried out in more than one way, it's important that you follow the exam instructions on what technique to demonstrate. For instance, as a CNA you might feed a patient who is in bed or who is seated in a chair. That's why the exam will specify such details. It's important that you know various techniques for accomplishing the same task because that knowledge may be tested in the written part of the CNA exam.

## Checkpoints for Different Skills

Although the skills tested in the practical part of the CNA exam are few, every skill has checkpoints which the test proctor will use to rate how you have performed. Once the test is over, your proctor will enter his or her observations into a computer, where a Prometric system will determine your results.

You can expect to receive your CNA exam results on the same day you take the exam, unless there is a technology-related glitch. In case there is a problem and you don't receive your results on the exam day, you can access the results online. The testing center will provide you with information on how to do this.

When you take the practical part of the CNA exam, you will receive instructions pertaining to individual skills, and you will also be given related checkpoints. In short, it will be made clear to you what the evaluator will be looking for. For example, in the description given in your instructions, you will be informed if you are expected to use a mannequin or a real person to play the part of a resident receiving care.

If a real person is to going to play the role of a resident receiving care, often one of the CNA exam candidates will play the part. But don't be surprised if the proctor decides to play the part of the resident because that does happen occasionally.

As you wait for your exam to begin, you will be provided with general instructions to read. These instructions are basic rules you should follow in the clinical skills test. Read these carefully. You may find, for example, instructions on what to do if you find it necessary to correct a mistake you made in a particular skill you were demonstrating.

In case you want to see these general instructions beforehand, log onto www.prometric.com/nurseaide and check the instructions under your state. In fact, it's advisable to familiarize yourself with these general instructions before the day of the exam.

Other checkpoints include asking a resident if he or she has any preferences as you provide care. The proctor will be interested to see if you involve the resident as you carry out your task and show respect by asking the resident about his or her preference. You'll also be assessed to see if you ask the resident about his or her comfort or personal needs as you provide care.

Another checkpoint is adherence to standard precautions and measures to ensure control of infection. Additionally, your skills in ensuring safety for the resident will be checked, such as when you help a resident use a bedpan.

## What to Do Once in the Exam Room

Once you have entered the room where you will be tested, you will be made familiar with the setting so that you know the exact location of the equipment required for the exam and also where the supplies have been placed. The exam room is normally set up in a manner that resembles an actual resident's room.

For example, items like toothbrushes and toothpaste, bedpans and basins will be placed inside the cabinet by the bed the same way they would be in a resident's room.

As you take the clinical skills test, keep in mind the expectations, which are that you will perform the skills the same way they are actually practiced in a nursing facility. Note that your proctor is not permitted to answer questions about techniques for performing any skills.

# Specific Abilities Evaluated

In order for you to score well on the exam, you need to demonstrate that you can execute the most important skills when it comes to providing personal care to patients. Among those skills is handwashing.

### *Skill in Handwashing*

Handwashing skills are so important that they are tested and scored in all states which administer CNA certification exams. You will be tested not only on how you wash your hands but on how long you wash them for.

During the exam you should not expect to receive instructions on when to wash your hands, because you should already know you must wash them before touching a resident. The proctor will be watching how skilled you are at properly washing your hands. In some states, such as Florida, a nurse will monitor your handwashing before you begin completing the test of your initial skill, and a different nurse will monitor your handwashing after completion of that initial skill.

When it's time to wash your hands, make sure that you use either warm or cold running water. Begin by wetting your hands and then turn off the faucet before applying soap to your hands.

After you have lathered your wet hands generously, rub them together so they are well covered with soap. You need to particularly check that the back area of your hands is well lathered, and also check in between your fingers and the spaces under your fingernails. Next, scrub your hands thoroughly for half a minute, or a minimum of 20 seconds.

To ensure you clean all spaces properly, interlock your fingers every now and then as you scrub. You should also ensure you scrub the back parts of your fingers thoroughly, along with your fingertips, thumbs and wrists.

Since it may not be convenient for you to keep checking your watch during the handwashing test, make sure that before the test you come up with a technique to accurately count the seconds. You might choose a song or chorus to hum silently, or a poem that lasts 20 seconds or so while you recite it to yourself.

After thoroughly scrubbing, rinse your hands using clean running water. Finally, use a clean towel to dry your hands or alternatively, air-dry them.

*General Handwashing Tips*

(a)    Don't substitute handwashing with hand sanitizers during the exam or at other times. Sanitizers are meant as an addition to handwashing and not as a replacement. Furthermore, too much reliance on sanitizers can dry your skin because sanitizers often have alcohol in them.

(b)    If you are taking care of a child and need to wash his or her hands, you may want to sing a 30-second song to get the child into the habit of washing his or her hands for the duration of the song. That way you will not only clean the child's hands appropriately but you will also be helping the child learn proper handwashing technique.

Additionally, make sure to always wash your hands:

(c)    Before and after eating

(d)    After being outdoors

(e)    After using the toilet

(f)    After sneezing or coughing

(g)    After you've been with someone ill.

Getting into the habit of handwashing keeps you healthy and prevents the transfer of disease-causing microorganisms from one person or place to another.

### Skill in Indirect Patient Care

CNAs are expected to also be able to provide care to patients in an indirect manner.

Direct patient care is when you are in one-on-one contact with the patient, such as when you're cleaning a wound. Indirect patient care does not involve one-on-one contact. If a patient is hard of hearing and you advise family members to speak at a certain volume, that's indirect care. Another example is shutting the window in the patient's room to protect that patient from the cold.

### Skill in Taking a Patient's Vital Signs

CNAs are expected to be skilled in measuring and recording the blood pressure of a patient, body temperature, pulse and respiration rate. For each of these vital signs, the CNA is expected to know the optimal level or count that is considered normal, the acceptable range and when a level or count is too high or too low.

In the same vein, CNAs are expected to know the effect on a patient when these measurements rise above normal range or drop below normal range. When a nurse instructs a CNA to carry out a task owing to a discrepancy in a patient's vital signs, the CNA is expected to have an idea what is expected. For instance, a CNA is expected to know to use a warm, wet cloth on a patient's forehead when his or her temperature is higher than normal.

### Skills in Testing a Patient's Range of Motion

CNAs are expected to be able to test a patient's range of motion (ROM) in a passive manner. Such motions target the patient's shoulders and elbows as well as wrists, ankles, knees and hips.

ROM measures how well a patient can move a particular joint or body part. Usually ROM is assessed during physical therapy. Sometimes ROM is also performed to assess a patient's strength, flexibility or balance.

### Skill in Using a Gait Belt

Medical institutions provide gait belts to help transfer patients who have problems walking from their beds to wheelchairs. Gait belts also help when assisting a patient to sit down, stand up or walk around. The gait belt is secured along the patient's waist and allows a CNA to grasp it, making it easier to assist the patient with movements. The proctor will evaluate how appropriately you use the gait belt.

For starters, the proctor will check how you use the gait belt and how you remove it from a resident's waist without causing any harm. For example, the proctor will notice any inappropriate pulling that you do on the belt as the resident sits down in a chair after a walk.

How you position the resident in the chair before you leave is important and will be evaluated to see if you align the body properly and seat the resident's hips properly against the back of the chair.

### Skill in Positioning Patients

There are different positions patients are expected to be placed in as physicians and nurses carry out procedures, or as CNAs carry out certain tasks such as giving back massages. Common positions include the supine position, the prone position, lateral position, Fowler's position and Sims position. You may be tested on some of these positions.

### Skill in Feeding Patients

Since CNAs often work with patients who are weak, old or incapacitated, they are expected to know how to feed them and also how to correctly measure food and fluids.

You may be tested in your skills in this area as well as in accurately recording a patient's intake.

CNAs are expected to know how to use different feeding positions for individual patients depending on their respective challenges.

### Skill in Providing Oral Care

A CNA should be able to demonstrate skills in providing oral care to patients, mostly elderly individuals, who wear dentures. They should also be able to demonstrate skills in providing oral care to unconscious patients. This is of fundamental importance because unconscious patients are always at a higher risk of aspiration. CNAs should also be able to assist conscious patients who have medical conditions that hinder their ability to brush their teeth independently.

### Skill in Providing Care for Hand, Nails and Feet

The hands, nails and feet require meticulously hygiene to prevent bacterial infections. Hands are especially important with regards to hygiene, and CNAs need to ensure patients are taught proper hygiene techniques and assisted as necessary.

### Skill in Providing Perineal Care

CNAs are expected to be skilled in assisting patients afflicted by diseases affecting the urinary tract, bladder and kidneys. This kind of care is termed 'perineal care' and sometimes is referred to as 'peri care.'

Literally speaking, perineal care is simply the washing of a patient's genitals and anal region. CNAs should expect to provide this care on a regular basis, sometimes during a patient's a bath. However, owing to the nature of a patient's illness, some individuals may require frequent perineal care that is not linked to bathing time. One of the major reasons CNAs are expected to be skilled in perineal care is that it protects patients from skin breaking down around the perineal region, which might in turn lead to infection. Careful perineal care also prevents itching, burning and the development of foul odors.

### Skill in Providing Bathing Care

CNAs are expected to assist patients with limited mobility to bathe, though sometimes the help required is only partial. They are also required to give bed baths to bedridden patients.

You should know the recommended sequence for bathing a patient. This involves starting with the areas of the body that are considered least dirty, and ending with those considered most dirty. This is precautionary as the sequence minimizes the chances of spreading bacteria and any other disease-causing microorganisms from one part of the body to others.

## Skill in Providing Dressing Assistance

Among the duties entrusted to CNAs is assisting patients to dress whose arms are weak following stroke, injury or other medical issues. You can expect to be tested on skills relating to the process of dressing a patient who is completely or partially dependent, and part of the behavior tested is how polite you are to the patient and whether or not you keep talking to ensure patients feel comfortable as you attend to them.

This is an area where you will certainly be tested on your handwashing hygiene because you will need to wash your hands thoroughly before starting to assist the patient. You will also be observed to see whether you begin by undressing the part of the patient that is weakest. The proctor will observe whether you are making any effort to teach the patient how to try to dress him or herself. You could also be tested on how close to a patient you place clean clothes.

## Skill in Providing Toileting Assistance

CNAs are expected to demonstrate skills in assisting patients who are too weak or incapacitated to use the toilet independently. Besides the fundamental handwashing skills, the proctor will expect to see if you:

- Know how to lower a patient's bed
- position the patient in the required supine position
- put the patient's bedpan close enough
- assist the patient to move some distance from the bed as needed
- position the bedpan appropriately beneath the buttocks
- and all other skills associated with toileting care.

During the exam, the part of a resident needing toileting assistance will be acted out by someone who wears a hospital gown. For testing purposes, you should pretend you are assisting a resident who has no underwear on as you demonstrate the use of the bedpan.

The proctor will check whether you greet the resident on arrival, introduce yourself and address him or her by name. Another checkpoint is whether you explain the caregiving procedure to the patient in advance and also during the process.

You are expected to put a protective pad underneath a resident's buttocks and on top of the bed's lower sheet before proceeding to the second step where you place the bedpan on the pad for the resident to use.

You will also be required to demonstrate that you are skilled in cleaning a patient well enough to prevent infection, and also will be observed on your knowledge of properly disposing of the contents of the bedpan.

The bedpan should be positioned underneath the resident with consideration as to its shape. Furthermore, the way you position the bedpan should make it easy to be removed. The proctor will want to see how you raise the head of the bed once you have positioned the resident on the bedpan, and also how you lower it to remove the used bedpan.

It is expected that you will ask the resident to ring the bell to call you once he or she is through emptying his or her bladder and bowels.

The proctor will check whether you remember to put the toilet paper somewhere the resident can reach it. You will be expected to wear gloves as you remove the bedpan after use, and to keep them on as you empty the bedpan. You will also be monitored on whether you follow procedure by immediately cleaning the bedpan while you have your gloves on.

The bedpan contents are expected to be emptied in the toilet, and the proctor will note whether you do so and then rinse the bedpan before drying it. You are also expected to give the resident a damp washcloth and a hand wipe after he or she uses the bedpan.

To complete the procedure, make sure you put the bedpan back in its place, return the toilet paper to its usual location, place any soiled linen in the hamper and dispose of any trash.

### Skill in Monitoring & Measuring Urine

You could be tested on how skilled you are in providing catheter care to patients. You should be able to demonstrate that you can record urine output with accuracy. These skills are particularly important when taking care of patients with urinary issues or other kidney-related problems.

### Skill in Changing Linen in an Occupied Bed

Sometimes a CNA needs to change bedsheets while a patient is still occupying the bed, particularly if a patient has limited mobility. You should therefore be able to demonstrate the best procedure to follow in removing the dirty linen and replacing it with clean linen without interfering with the welfare and comfort of the patient.

For starters, you need to let the patient occupying the bed know you are there to change the sheets. Then remove the top blanket, followed by the top sheet. Where you place the bedding you intend to reuse, such as the top blanket, and the bed linen you don't intend to reuse, such as sheets, is important. You are also expected to demonstrate you know how to roll the patient carefully in order to change the sheets under his or her body. You'll also be observed on how you change a pillow cover when the pillow is still being used by a patient.

# Test 1: Questions

(1) Every CNA is aware that it's not her or his duty to _____.

(A) Help a resident take a bath

(B) Administer medication

(C) Keep a resident's room clean

(D) Apply an ice pack

(2) Identify the option below that exemplifies patient battery.

(A) The CNA bathes the patient without that resident's permission

(B) The CNA seeks prior permission to touch the patient when that resident needs assistance to visit the bathroom

(C) The CNA cleans the patient's glasses

(D) The CNA isolates the patient from other residents in a bid to punish him or her

(3) After seeing unexplained bruises on a patient, a CNA is suspicious that a particular resident is being abused. In addition, the resident refuses to answer the majority of questions asked and also refuses ADLs. What step would you advise the CNA to take in regards to the situation?

(A) The CNA should immediately report his or her own suspicions to a supervisor

(B) The CNA should immediately alert the nurse who handles the patient's direct care about the bruises

(C) The CNA should be persistent in asking the resident who the abuser is

(D) The CNA should be patient and wait for additional proof of abuse

(4) Which of the options below exemplifies MRSA?

(A) A bacterial strain that is easily treated with antibiotics

(B) A mnemonic that easily reminds you how to act if a fire erupts in a facility you are in

(C) Activities that residents are expected to engage in so as to remain safe

(D) A drug-resistant bacterial strain which antibiotics cannot easily treat


(5) Which of the options below rates highest as far as prevention of infection is concerned?

(A) Using hand sanitizer after working with a patient

(B) Wearing gloves whenever there is a chance of coming into contact with someone's bodily fluids

(C) Washing your hands frequently

(D) Relying on standard precautions when caring for patients


(6) When giving a patient a bath, a CNA should always _____.

(A) Use mostly cool water in order to improve the patient's blood circulation

(B) Allow the patient to participate in the care being provided so as to encourage the patient to feel more independent

(C) Clean the patient's perineal region before helping the patient clean his or her own face

(D) Perform all care for the patient so the patient is able to conserve his or her energy

(7) When a CNA is caring for a resident, which of the options listed below is best where a resident's skin is concerned?

(A) The CNA notices there is an area of the resident's sacrum that is red and non-blanchable and reports it to the patient's nurse

(B) The CNA decides not to start any care associated with the perineal area until another member of staff is present

(C) The CNA carefully puts talcum powder under the patient's abdominal folds

(D) The CNA applies ointment to the patient as prescribed


(8) A CNA must always check for _____ within a patient's care plan before shaving the resident.

(A) Any history of heart problems

(B) Specific instructions on shaving when a patient has a blood-clotting problem

(C) Accessibility to a razor brought from home for the resident

(D) Any record of the patient having refused ADLs in the past


(9) Which of the options below is a symptom of fecal impaction?

(A) A lot of flatulence

(B) Dark urine

(C) Abdominal pain

(D) Watery stool leakage

(10) The term 'dyspnea' is used in reference to difficulty _____

(A) Urinating

(B) Defecating

(C) Breathing

(D) Swallowing


(11) Which of the options below is a fact about residents with Alzheimer's disease?

(A) There is no way residents with Alzheimer's can be reoriented as they are bound to forget soon

(B) It's best if residents with Alzheimer's maintain a routine so as to reduce the chances of confusion and overstimulation

(C) Confusion is normal for Alzheimer's patients, but hallucinations are not

(D) The appetite of a person with Alzheimer's increases with time as the disease progresses


(12) When a bed is already occupied, you should remember that _____.

(A) Until you finish remaking the bed, you should place the dirty linen right on the floor

(B) You should not raise the bed rails unless it becomes really necessary

(C) You should not miter the corners of the fresh sheets

(D) It's important to lower the bed as far down as possible once you are through with the procedure

(13)  A CNA should make a point of reporting to the nurse if a patient's pulse rate is _____.

(A) 98

(B) 45

(C) 64

(D) 82


(14)  Which of the following is a sign of hypoglycemia?

(A) Polyuria

(B) Skin that is dry and hot

(C) Sweating

(D) Tachycardia


(15)  Which of the following statements is true when working with hard-of-hearing residents?

(A) It's important that you speak slowly and clearly

(B) It's important that you speak in a high pitch

(C) It's preferable that you use written words to communicate rather than speak

(D) It's important that you involve family members so that they can understand what you are telling the hearing impaired resident

(16)  What option listed below represents the High Fowler position?

(A) The patient sits upright while his or her bed is at a right angle or at 90°

(B) The patient sits slumped a little to the left as his or her bed is positioned at an angle of 30°

(C) The patient's feet are propped up while his or her bed is at an angle of 60°

(D) The patient is in a prone position with his or her stomach touching the bed and should remain in that position for 20 minutes before feeding time

(17)  What equipment should a CNA use when it's time to change an incontinent patient's clothes?

(A) An N-95 mask

(B) A gown and gloves

(C) A gown and mask

(D) A pair of gloves, a gown and a mask

(18)  If a resident has an infection, the CNA may observe _____.

(A) Skin pallor

(B) Sudden confusion

(C) Tented skin

(D) Aphasia

(19)  What does 'NPO' stand for?

(A) Strictly bedrest

(B) Diet in liquid form

(C) Do not take oral temperature

(D) Nothing by mouth


(20)  If a CNA finds that a diabetic patient _____, he or she must inform the nurse as soon as possible.

(A) Fails to eat anything at lunchtime

(B) Insists on combing his hair at odd times

(C) Reports feeling numb in the feet at times

(D) Refuses to finish writing a will he or she has started


(21)  As a CNA, how often should you turn your patients?

(A) Every eight hours

(B) Every hour

(C) Every two hours

(D) Every six hours

(22) Which of the following is a CNA likely to use when she or he wants to measure a patient's pulse?

(A) Brachial

(B) Radial

(C) Femoral

(D) Popliteal


(23) A CNA is in the dining hall with residents, helping them eat. All of a sudden one of the residents stands up and starts to clutch his throat as he releases a silent cough. What action should the CNA take first?

(A) Immediately call 911

(B) Immediately start the Heimlich maneuver

(C) Ask the resident if he is choking

(D) Immediately begin to administer CPR


(24) A client arrives at a facility and is shown a room that she will be sharing with a resident who has been at the facility for a year. When the newly arrived client goes to the bathroom, the established resident leans over and inquires, "Why is this new lady here? Is she sick?" The answer the CNA should give is _____.

(A) "You should mind your own business."

(B) "I'm afraid that information is confidential and so I cannot tell you."

(C) "She has the same problem you have."

(D) "I'll check her chart and then tell you."

(25) After an Alzheimer's patient has had breakfast it is important to provide support for the normal function of the gastrointestinal tract by _____.

(A) Recording the patient's intake and output

(B) Helping the patient go to the bathroom

(C) Helping the patient brush his teeth

(D) Assisting the patient in calling a member of his family

(26) A resident with type 2 diabetes asks a CNA to cut her toenails. Which of the actions listed below should the CNA take?

(A) Make a point of checking the patient's blood sugar level before trimming the nails

(B) Give the patient a safety clipper to use

(C) Read the patient's chart to see what the doctor has ordered with regard to trimming of nails

(D) Report the nail trimming request to a nurse

(27) To prevent insomnia, a CNA should _____.

(A) Recommend patients eat at least one apple each day

(B) Encourage patients to take regular walks around the residential facility

(C) Encourage patients to sleep all day

(D) Encourage patients to take several naps a day

(28) A CNA takes an elderly resident's temperature. The thermometer reads 100.6°F, and the resident tells the CNA he has just sipped some hot tea. The CNA should _____.

(A) Wait for a minimum of 15 minutes and then take the resident's temperature again

(B) Admonish the resident for drinking hot tea before having his temperature taken

(C) Take the patient's axillary temperature as an alternative

(D) Make a recording on the patient's chart of the 100.6°F temperature

(29) A CNA is caring for a patient who has chronic 'foot drop.' What device is the CNA likely to find in such a patient's room?

(A) A mechanical lift

(B) Two additional pillows

(C) A pair of positioning boots

(D) A wedge

(30) One of the residents at a health care facility reports feeling dizzy. The CNA takes the resident's heart rate and it's 82/43. What should the CNA do?

(A) Record the vital signs in the resident's chart

(B) Report the resident's heart rate to a nurse

(C) Take the resident's pulse rate

(D) Advise the resident to begin drinking plenty of fluids

(31) 'Abduction' is a term used in motion range to mean _____.

(A) Moving the extremity above the person's body

(B) Moving the extremity below the person's body

(C) Making the extremity toward the person's body

(D) Moving the extremity away from the person's body


(32) Which of the following is a way of addressing the spiritual needs of a client?

(A) Asking the client the reason he or she follows a particular faith

(B) Assisting the client to get to the chapel at the facility every Sunday

(C) Handling any religious objects in the client's room the same way other objects are handled

(D) Providing the client with a towel, soap and clean, warm water every Sunday


(33) When lifting a client, which of the following is best for appropriate mechanics of the body?

(A) Ensuring the client's knees are bent

(B) Ensuring the client's spine is curved

(C) Ensuring the client is bent at the waist

(D) Avoiding getting assistance from anyone else

(34)  Which of the following options suggests a client has hepatitis?

(A) Hyperglycemia

(B) Jaundice

(C) Hypotension

(D) Hypertension


(35)  If you notice a client is confused, the best action to take is _____.

(A) Ask what his or her name is

(B) Keep checking the client's blood glucose on an hourly basis

(C) Keep reorienting the client with mementos belonging to his or her family, calendars or the clock

(D) Keep the client confined in his or her room


(36)  Which of the following clients is likely to need hospice care?

(A) A client who has diabetes

(B) A client who has cancer

(C) A client who has kidney disease

(D) A client who has a terminal disease


(37)  Cheyne-Stokes respirations are known to occur in clients who _____.

(A) Are recovering from asthmatic attacks

(B) Are unconscious

(C) Are near death

(D) Are known to have chronic respiratory issues

(38)     If a resident has a panic attack, the CNA should immediately _____.

(A) Encourage the resident to express his or her feelings in words

(B) Instruct the resident to breathe slowly and deeply

(C) Ask the resident what caused the panic attack

(D) Distract the resident


(39)  Which of the following is an example of orthopneic positioning?

(A) A resident walking with the help of a cane

(B) A resident seated on one side of the bed while leaning forward over a table

(C) A resident seated upright in a chair

(D) A resident lying on his or stomach with his or her head turned to the side


(40)  A resident wants to choose some potassium-rich food items to incorporate into her breakfast. Which of the following foods is richest in potassium?

(A) Cantaloupe

(B) Toast

(C) Strawberries

(D) Eggs

(41)  When assisting a client who has weakness on the left side owing to CVA, how should the CNA position the client's cane?

(A) To the left of the client

(B) Some distance from the client

(C) To the right of the client

(D) Immediately in front of the client


(42)  A patient should be given CPR when _____.

(A) There is no breathing or pulse detected in the patient

(B) The patient is unconscious

(C) The patient appears to be choking

(D) The patient is not breathing though a pulse can be felt


(43)  A CNA enters a patient's room and finds the trash can has a fire burning inside it. What action should the CNA immediately take?

(A) Call a nurse to come help

(B) Reach for the facility's fire alarm

(C) Remove the patient from the room

(D) Put out the fire

(44) 'Log rolling' is a medical technique often used when a patient has been diagnosed with _____.

(A) Psychosis

(B) Spinal cord injury

(C) Right-arm cellulitis

(D) Left tibial fracture


(45) Patients who habitually refuse to go to the bathroom are putting themselves at risk of developing _____.

(A) Incontinence

(B) Low appetite

(C) Constipation

(D) Insomnia


(46) Which of the following is part of the normal grieving process?

(A) Complicated grieving

(B) Anticipatory grieving

(C) Inhibited grieving

(D) Unresolved grieving

(47) Which of the following is not permitted when a patient is on a clear liquid diet?

(A) Tea

(B) Water

(C) Orange juice with pulp

(D) Coffee


(48) The doctor orders twice daily ambulation of a client who has a Foley catheter. The CNA should _____ before starting to ambulate the client.

(A) Request that the nurse confirm the order

(B) Ensure the bag is raised above the level of the client's bladder

(C) Ensure the bag is positioned below the level of the client's bladder

(D) Ensure the client covers the bag using a pillow


(49) When is it necessary to restrain a patient?

(A) Under orders from a physician

(B) When restraints are of a physical nature

(C) When approved by the nurse in charge

(D) When approved by the hospital's administrator

(50) You have a patient who has just eaten a bagel and consumed a big glass of apple juice. What is the best way to record the patient's fluid intake?

(A) 120 cc

(B) 480 cc

(C) 480 ml

(D) 120 ml


(51) There is a patient in the unit whom the doctor has put on airborne precautions because of suspicion of tuberculosis. The doctor has ordered that specimens of the patient's sputum be taken so he can then have them analyzed. What is the appropriate time of the day for the CNA to collect the specimens on a daily basis?

(A) Before the patient eats

(B) After the patient eats

(C) Early in the morning before the patient has done anything else

(D) Late in the evening just before the patient retires to bed


(52) If a CNA enters a patient's room and finds him masturbating, which of the following is the best action to take?

(A) Immediately leave the patient's room to accord him privacy

(B) Ask the patient why he is doing it

(C) Admonish the patient and let him know it's a shameful thing to do

(D) Report what you saw to the nurse

(53) A CNA is dealing with a patient who is yelling, screaming and trying to bite her. What action should the CNA take?

(A) Switch on the TV to distract the patient

(B) Speak authoritatively but calmly to the patient

(C) Only provide the patient with critical care

(D) Restrain the patient for his or her own safety


(54) A terminally ill client tells the CNA he has gotten into the habit of praying every night and believes God is going to forgive him. Which of the following stages of grief is the patient going through?

(A) Denial

(B) Bargaining

(C) Acceptance

(D) Anger


(55) A CNA wants to help a patient who has been immobilized by disease to leave the bed and move to a chair. Which of the following is the best equipment for the CNA to use?

(A) A transfer belt

(B) A sheet

(C) A Hoyer lift

(D) Wrist restraints

(56) A CNA is about to give a patient a bath just before bedtime. However, the CNA notices the patient has a Foley catheter in place, which means she needs to secure it to ensure there is no risk of it being pulled out when the patient is being bathed. Where should the CNA secure the catheter?

(A) To one of the patient's bedsheets

(B) To the patient's lateral thigh

(C) To the patient's bed

(D) To the patient's thigh

(57) A patient who has just received terrible news that his wife has died is distraught as he tells the CNA he can't believe what he has just been told. He tells the CNA that he can't see how he can live without his wife. Which of the following is the best response from the CNA?

(A) I know you are in real pain. I'll stay here and keep you company.

(B) Soon or later everyone will lose a loved one.

(C) You need time to cope with your loss.

(D) Do you have any children?

(58) A CNA is helping a patient to bathe, and that patient has recently suffered a stroke on his right side. In order to enhance the patient's independence, the CNA should _____.

(A) Ask what role he wants to play in the bathing process

(B) Encourage the patient to try and bathe himself as best as he can

(C) Permit the patient to participate in bathing himself as much as possible

(D) Bathe the patient yourself so he can conserve all his energy

(59) A patient has burned his leg after accidentally pouring some hot soup on it. The skin is red and blistered. According to the CNA, this is a case of _____.

(A) Superficial burn

(B) Total thickness burn

(C) Partial thickness burn

(D) Serious burn


(60) The CNA notices a client has experienced no bowel movements for four days. Which procedure listed below would be most beneficial to the client?

(A) Catheterization

(B) A colonoscopy

(C) An enema

(D) An endoscopy

# Test 1: Answers & Explanations

(1) Every CNA is aware that it is not her or his duty as a CNA to _____.

The correct answer is: (B) administer medication.

CNAs are not permitted to administer medication. It's not part of their responsibilities. Staff permitted to administer medication includes RNs and LPNs. In the USA and Canada, an LPN is expected to provide care to injured patients, but LPNs also care for the disabled, ill or convalescent. LPNs are individually responsible for whatever actions they take in treating patients. In some US states such as California and Texas, LPNs are known as LVNs, which stands for Licensed Vocational Nurses. To become an LPN, one needs to train for two years in the US. In Canada training takes two to three years after completing a secondary school course, and passing the Canadian Practical Nurse Registration Exam is also a requirement.

(2)   Identify the option below that exemplifies patient battery.

The correct answer is: (A) The CNA bathes the patient without that resident's permission.

If a CNA bathes a patient before obtaining permission first, it's considered battery. Isolating the patient from the rest of the residents exemplifies involuntary seclusion. Battery is when a person intentionally, offensively and possibly injuriously touches a person without the affected individual giving consent.

Battery should not be confused with assault, which also sometimes happens in nursing homes. Examples of assault by CNAs include pretending to hit a patient or issuing verbal threats. One difference between battery and assault is that in battery you can hurt someone without warning them first or making them fearful. Like in this question, the CNA could just enter the patient's room and begin undressing him or her for a bath without prior warning.

(3)    After seeing unexplained bruises on a patient, a CNA is suspicious that a particular resident is being abused. In addition, the resident refuses to answer the majority of questions asked and also refuses ADLs. What step would you advise the CNA to take in regards to the situation?

The correct answer is: (A) The CNA should immediately report his or her suspicions to a supervisor.

If anyone, including a CNA, notices or is suspicious of patient abuse, they should report their observations to their immediate supervisor as soon as possible. Cases of abuse require more action than a CNA is authorized to take, and so the only way to solve the problem is by reporting it to someone with more authority to address such matters. While it is a good idea to notify the nurse offering direct care to the affected patient about the bruising you have observed, the nurse may focus on how to heal the bruises but may take a while to realize there is a bigger problem than the current bruises. In the meantime, the abuse could continue.

(4)    Which of the options below exemplifies MRSA?

The correct answer is: (D) A drug-resistant bacterial strain which antibiotics cannot easily treat.

Methicillin-Resistant Staphylococcus Aureus (MRSA) is a bacterial strain known for its resistance to most antibiotics including penicillin, methicillin, amoxicillin and oxacillin.

The staphylococcus aureus bacterium resides in a person's nose or skin. Even with the resistance some of these bacteria develop, the good news is that their spread is greatly curtailed by use of germ-destroying soaps and germ-destroying ointments.

(5)    Which of the options below rates highest as far as prevention of infection is concerned?

Option (C), making sure to wash your hands frequently, constitutes the best precautionary measure you can take. The other options besides (C) only offer supportive measures. Even when the CNA is going to wear gloves or has just used gloves, handwashing should not be ignored.

(6)    When giving a patient a bath, a CNA should always _____.

The correct answer is: (B) Allow the patient to participate in the care being provided so as to encourage him or her to feel more independent.

As you let the patient participate in bathing or in his or her care in general, you help boost self-confidence. The other answer options are completely wrong. For one, using cool water is not recommended as it is not normally as comfortable as warm water. And cleaning the patient's perineal region before cleaning the face is completely inappropriate.

(7)    When a CNA is caring for a resident, which of the options listed below is best if were a resident's skin is concerned?

The correct answer is: (A) The CNA notices there is an area of the resident's sacrum that is red and non-blanchable and reports it to the patient's nurse.

The CNA is always expected to report any redness on a patient's skin to the nurse. Even if the CNA may have an idea what the reddened pressure spots are, he or she must still report the redness to the nurse, who can then determine the appropriate course of action.
A CNA is not mandated to apply prescription ointment on a patient, and talcum powder is not recommended for a patient's skin care. When it is time to provide perineal care to a patient, one CNA is all that is needed.

(8)    A CNA must always check for _____ within a patient's care plan before shaving the resident.

The correct answer is: (B) Specific instructions on shaving when a patient has a blood-clotting problem.

Before shaving a patient, the CNA needs to go through the patient's care plan to see if there is any record of the patient having blood-clotting problems, and what it says about handling his shaving. It is especially important to learn from the care plan if it is preferable to use an electric razor on a resident as opposed to a traditional one.

(9)    Which of the options below is a symptom of fecal impaction?

The correct answer is: (D) Watery stool leakage.

When a person has a fecal blockage, usually watery stool leaks around that blockage. Such leakage is a sign there is a bowel obstruction. Often when people have fecal impaction, they will have gone several days without a bowel movement, and in the meantime a mass of hard stool will have formed within the colon or rectum. Many times people with fecal impaction will have had prior problems with bowel movements and will have regularly used laxatives.


(10)  The term 'dyspnea' is used in reference to difficulty _____

The correct answer is: (C) Breathing.

The term 'dyspnea' is a medical term used in reference to difficulty in breathing whether mild and temporary or serious and long-lasting. There are different factors that can lead to dyspnea, including a high elevation environment or a person having overexerted himself or herself. The term 'dyspnea' can be used when a person feels like he or she is suffocating, is experiencing tightness in the chest, has labored breathing and palpitations or is wheezing and/or coughing.


(11)   Which of the options below is a fact about residents with Alzheimer's disease?

(E) The correct answer is: (B) It's best if residents with Alzheimer's maintain a routine so as to reduce the chances of confusion and overstimulation.

When it comes to Alzheimer's patients a standard routine reduces incidences of confusion. As for the other answer options, they are incorrect because for starters, it is both possible and advisable to reorient a person with Alzheimer's. Hallucinations do occur and are usually part of the disease. The appetite of someone with Alzheimer's does not increase as the disease progresses; it actually decreases.

(12)  When a bed is already occupied, you should remember that _____.

The correct answer is: (D) It's important to lower the bed as far down as possible once you are through with the procedure.

The reason it's important to lower the bed as far as possible is for the safety of the patient. The other options are incorrect. Placing soiled bedding on the floor is highly discouraged. It's recommended that bed rails be kept raised and that the corners of the bedsheets be mitered. To miter a corner means to fold it at right angles. This makes the patient more comfortable as the bed corners are left smooth and neat.

(13)  A CNA should make a point of reporting to the nurse if a patient's pulse rate is _____.

The correct answer is: (B) 45.

If a pulse rate is 45, a CNA should report that to a nurse. A pulse rate of 45 is unsafe. A normal range of pulse rate is from 60 up to 100. Having a heart rate that is slow in an abnormal way, also known as bradycardia, is unhealthy and involves the heart beating fewer than 60 times per minute.

(14)  Which of the following is a sign of hypoglycemia?

The correct answer is: (C) sweating.

The term 'hypoglycemia' is used in reference to a situation where the level of glucose in a person's bloodstream is abnormally low. In this question, sweating is the correct answer as it is among the signs of hypoglycemia. Tremors and confusion are other signs of hypoglycemia, as are trembling and nausea, as well as a racing heart. In serious cases of hypoglycemia, a person can fall into a coma or even die. There are varying causes of hypoglycemia but mostly it occurs when someone has reacted to a type of medication like insulin, which is what diabetics use for treatment when their blood sugar level is high.

(15)  Which of the following statements is true when working with hard-of-hearing residents?

The correct answer is: (A) It's important that you speak slowly and clearly.

People trying to communicate with a person who is hard of hearing are always advised to speak as slowly and clearly as possible, as this helps that person to follow what you are trying to say. In addition to facing the person with a hearing impairment when speaking, you also need to make eye contact as you talk. At the same time, try as much as possible to talk to the patient in a location that does not have background noise. When dealing with someone who is hearing impaired, make repeating yourself and rephrasing what you have said part of normal conversation.

(16)  What option listed below represents the High Fowler position?

The correct answer is: (A) The patient sits upright while his or her bed is at a right angle or at 90°.

The High Fowler position refers to a patient being seated upright at 90°. Mostly such cases will be in a hospital setting, and the upper body of the patient is between 60° and 90° relative to the patient's lower part of the body. It is standard practice for nurses to put patients who have breathing challenges in the High Fowler position.

(17)  What equipment should a CNA use when it's time to change an incontinent patient's clothes?

The correct answer is: (B) A gown and gloves.

Incontinence is when a patience does not have voluntary control of urination, defecation or both. For protection, a CNA should always wear a pair of gloves as well as a gown when changing an incontinent patient's clothing. Urinary incontinence is when a person's urine leaks involuntarily or a patient urinates without intending to. Patients with anal incontinence normally have lost any control of their sphincter, where sphincter means the muscle that surrounds the concerned openings, whether it is the person's anus, opening to the stomach or other such areas.

(18)  If a resident has an infection, the CNA may observe _____.

The correct answer is: (B) Sudden confusion.

Infection is one of the ailments that can make patients become confused all of a sudden, especially elderly patients. Tented skin cannot be relied upon as a sign of infection because for elderly patients tented skin is normal. Aphasia is a possible symptom of a stroke but not infection.


(19)  What does 'NPO' stand for?

The correct answer is: (D) Nothing by mouth.

When the doctor has given medical instructions and indicated 'NPO,' it means a patient should not be given anything through the mouth, whether drinks, food or medication. The term 'NPO' is an abbreviation for the Latin 'nil per os.' When NPO orders are issued pre-surgery, it means they should be adhered to six to 12 hours before surgery and for a period afterwards during recovering. Sometimes NPO orders are longer than 12 hours, especially in cases where medications have a long-acting period or where oral post-operative medications have been administered. Usually NPO with regards to food is longer than NPO with regards to liquids. This is because doctors are discouraged by the American Board of Anesthesiology from not allowing patients to drink for more than eight hours.


(20) If a CNA finds that a diabetic patient _____, he or she must inform the nurse as soon as possible.

The correct answer is: (A) Fails to eat anything at lunchtime.

It's important for diabetic patients to eat something on a regular basis because that ensures their level of blood sugar remains stable. Feeling numb in the feet at times is not unusual for diabetic patients. In fact, it's considered a usual side effect of the condition and is termed 'neuropathy.'

(21)  As a CNA, how often should you turn your patients?

The correct answer is: (C)  Every two hours.

To maintain the integrity of a patient's skin, a patient needs to be turned every two hours.


(22)  Which of the following is a CNA likely to use when she or he wants to acquire a patient's pulse?

The correct answer is: (B) Radial.

A CNA can most easily access the radial pulse, situated on the inside of the wrist close to the thumb. Note that for a pulse result to be valid, you need to count the heart rate for a period of at least 15 seconds. You may wish to count the heart rate for longer, such as 20 to 60 seconds. Longer is fine; shorter is not.


(23)  A CNA is in the dining hall with residents, helping them eat. All of a sudden one of the residents stands up and starts to clutch his throat as he releases a silent cough. What action should the CNA take first?

The correct answer is: (C) Ask the resident if he is choking.

The CNA needs to find out first if the resident is actually choking. If the resident gives a verbal answer, it means there is still some passage for air to get through the trachea. If the patient nods in response to the question, then the CNA should administer the Heimlich maneuver. It is important to note that anyone with the ability to speak or cough should not be subjected to the Heimlich maneuver.

(24) A client arrives at a facility and is shown a room that she will be sharing with a resident who has been at the facility for a year. When the newly arrived client goes to the bathroom, the established resident leans over and inquires, "Why is this new lady here? Is she sick?" The answer the CNA should give is _____.

The correct answer is: (B) "I'm afraid that information is confidential and so I cannot tell you."

As a CNA, you should always treat information pertaining to the health of the patient as confidential. As such, you should not disclose it even to fellow patients. That is the law according to the Health Insurance Portability and Accountability Act (HIPPA).

(25) After an Alzheimer's patient resident has had breakfast, it is important to provide support for the normal function of the gastrointestinal tract by _____.

The correct answer is: (B) Helping the patient go to the bathroom.

Very likely after the CNA helps the patient access the bathroom, the patient will have a bowel movement and that is great for supporting the health of the gastrointestinal tract.

(26) A resident with type 2 diabetes asks a CNA to cut her toenails. Which of the actions listed below should the CNA take?

The correct answer is: (C) Read the patient's chart to see what the doctor has ordered with regard to trimming of nails.

When a resident is diabetic, the doctor makes a point of writing down instructions meant particularly for that patient pertaining to the issue of trimming the nails. For that reason, the CNA is expected to read the patient's chart to see the recommendation the doctor has given in that regard.

(27) To prevent insomnia, a CNA should _____.

The correct answer is: (B) Encourage patients to take regular walks around the residential facility.

Patients who take walks within the residential facility during the day are likely to enjoy better quality sleep at night.

(28) A CNA takes an elderly resident's temperature. The thermometer reads 100.6°F, and the resident tells the CNA he has just sipped some hot tea. The CNA should

_____.

The correct answer is: (A) Wait for a minimum of 15 minutes and then take the resident's temperature again.

After 15 minutes following the sipping of hot tea, the mouth's temperature should return to normal. Taking an axillary temperature may not be very useful, particularly if the patient is elderly.

(29) A CNA is caring for a patient who has chronic 'foot drop.' What device is the CNA likely to find in such a patient's room?

The correct answer is: (C) A pair of positioning boots.

Positioning boots are meant to ensure the wearer does not suffer discomfort or develop contractures because the feet are dorsiflexed—bent so they face somewhat upwards. This applies mainly to limbs like someone's foot or hand. You can, for example, speak of bending a resident's foot dorsally.

The term 'foot drop' is used in reference to an abnormality in a person's gait where the forefoot drops because of a weakness, damage to the fibular nerve or irritation. Where the fibular nerve has been damaged, usually the sciatic nerve is also adversely affected. Some people also develop foot drop owing to muscle paralysis, mostly affecting the muscles of the lower leg's anterior part. It is worth keeping in mind that foot drop on its own not really a disease. Instead, it serves as a symptom of a bigger medical problem.

(30) One of the residents at a health care facility reports feeling dizzy. The CNA takes the resident's heart rate and it's 82/43. What should the CNA do?

The correct answer is: (B) Report the resident's heart rate to a nurse.

When a heart rate is 82/43, it is classified as symptomatic, and the CNA should report all such cases to the nurse so he or she can investigate why the heart rate has dropped so precipitously.

(31) 'Abduction' is a term used in ROM to mean _____.

The correct answer is: (D) Moving the extremity away from the person's body.

The use of the term 'abduct' means moving away from something, while the use of the term 'adduct' means moving closer or toward something. For example, if you move one of your legs away from the midline of your body, this action can be described as 'abduction.' If you did the opposite, the action would be termed 'adduction.'

(32) Which of the following is a way of addressing the spiritual needs of a client?

The correct answer is: (B) Assisting the client to get to the chapel at the facility every Sunday.

If you want to help address the client's spiritual needs, help them fulfill what they desire as far as their religion or faith is concerned. In this regard, assisting your client to the chapel on Sundays will be very helpful, as matters of faith are discussed and religious ceremonies are carried out in the chapel mainly on Sundays. You also should not handle religious items like other ordinary items as doing so is disrespectful to a client's faith and religious values. Good examples of such religious items include the Bible for Christians, the rosary for Catholics, the Koran for Muslims and the Vedas for Hindus.

(33) When lifting a client, which of following is best for appropriate mechanics of the body?

The correct answer is: (A) Ensuring the client's knees are bent.

(A) Is the only appropriate answer. Ignore the suggestion about bending the client's spine or waist. Also, whether you get someone else to assist you when lifting a client or not has no bearing in the patient's body mechanics as long as you ensure the client's knees are bent as the lifting takes place.

(34) Which of the following suggests a client has hepatitis?

The correct answer is: (B) Jaundice.

Jaundice, which manifests in a person's change of skin color to yellow, is a disease affecting the liver. Such a disease might be hepatitis.

(35) If you notice a client is confused, the best action to take is _____.

The correct answer is: (C) Keep reorienting the client with mementos belonging to family, calendars or the clock.

It's of utmost importance to reorient a confused client. Some actions, such as confining the client to his or her room, are bad for the client's health. In fact, confining the client to his or her room, or any other room alone, could end up causing agitation. Even asking such clients to state their name is not helpful and might just make them unnecessarily agitated. In any case, there is a great chance they may not recall their name.

(36) Which of the following clients is likely to need hospice care?

The correct answer is: (D) A client who has a terminal disease.

Often clients who have terminal illnesses prefer to receive hospice care whose aim is to relieve the clients of pain. Healthcare providers are aware the clients are unlikely to be healed, have exhausted all feasible treatments and are prepared to focus on making the clients comfortable in their last days. Hospice care also incorporates efforts to meet the emotional and spiritual needs of clients.

(37)   Cheyne-Stokes respirations are known to occur in clients who _____.

The correct answer is: (C) are near death.

Cheyne-Stokes respirations occur when breathing is labored and the pattern indicates an increase in respirations with some durations of apnea. If a resident unexpectedly begins to show these signs, it is imperative that the CNA report the case immediately to a nurse or doctor. The term 'apnea' is used to mean there is no breathing.

(38)  If a resident has a panic attack, the CNA should immediately _____.

The correct answer is: (B) instruct the resident to breathe slowly and deeply.

The first thing the CNA should do is ensure the client is comfortable and then instruct him or her to breathe as slowly and deeply as possibly. It is also helpful to get the resident to slowly count backwards from 100. The CNA should not bother to ask the resident about the cause of the panic attack or discuss it, because such a discussion is bound to make the resident very uncomfortable. Normally people with panic attacks dread any discussion about their unpleasant feelings and frustrations. Also, there is no need to inquire about the cause as at such times it is difficult to concentrate on anything but the symptoms being experienced.

(39)  Which of the following is an example of orthopneic positioning?

The correct answer is: (B) A resident seated on one side of the bed while leaning forward over a table.

An orthopneic position is one that makes it easier to breathe. Leaning forward while seated facilitates entry of air into a person's lungs. The term 'orthopneic' is derived from the word 'orthopnea,' which refers to the state of running out of breath when in a prone position, and it is known to stop when a person changes position to sitting or standing. It is important to note that although orthopnea should be immediately addressed, it's not a disease on its own, but rather a symptom of another serious health problem such as lung disease or heart failure. Luckily, once the patient sits up, normal breathing should resume relatively fast. Sometimes the breath shortness can be accompanied by pain within the chest or tightness. Another condition similar to orthopnea, paroxysmal nocturnal dyspnea is where the patient awakes with breathing difficulties a few hours after falling asleep.

(40) A resident wants to choose some potassium-rich food items to incorporate into her breakfast. Which of the following foods is richest in potassium?

The correct answer is: (A) cantaloupe.

Cantaloupe is a kind of round melon very rich in potassium. It has orange flesh and skin that looks ribbed. The European Cantaloupe is light green on the outside. These cantaloupes have a nice fragrance when ripe, and because of it the fruits are sometimes called 'muskmelons.' Ordinarily 'musk' refers to a strongly scented substance musk deer produce that is often used in perfumes. Some other foods known for their richness in potassium include bananas and vegetables that are leafy and dark green.

(41) When assisting a client who has weakness on the left side owing to CVA, how should the CNA position the client's cane?

The correct answer is: (C) to the right of the client.

The reason the CNA should position the client's cane to the right is that the right side is the client's stronger side, and so positioning the cane on that side means the client can easily use it for support, including providing support to the weak left side. CVA is short for 'Cerebrovascular Accident' and simply means a stroke, which is the medical condition where blood ceases to reach a particular part of the brain. Such interference with blood flow to the brain happens sometimes because there is a blocked vessel or a vessel ruptures.

(42) A patient should be given CPR when _____.

The correct answer is: (A) There is no breathing or pulse detected in the patient.

CPR is short for 'cardiopulmonary resuscitation' and is a procedure carried out on an emergency basis, where the person administering it combines compressions of the chest and artificial ventilation in a bid to ensure the patient's brain continues functioning till such a time as more advanced medical help arrives. By the time CPR stops, it is anticipated that the medical measures replacing it will be able to restore the patient's ability to breathe and spontaneously circulate blood. Examples of patients requiring CPR are those experiencing cardiac arrest.

(43) A CNA enters a patient's room and finds the trash can has a fire burning inside. What action should the CNA immediately take?

The correct answer is: (C) Remove the patient from the room.

It is important that the CNA remove the patient from the room immediately and then other emergency steps can follow. Use the acronym 'RACE' to remember what to do during such a situation: Remove, Alarm, Contain, Extinguish.

(44) 'Log rolling' is a medical technique often used when a patient has been diagnosed with _____.

The correct answer is: (B) Spinal Cord Injury.

The log-rolling technique helps to avoid inflicting more damage on an already injured spinal cord by ensuring a patient's legs do not cross over his or her midline during a twisting movement.

(45) Patients who habitually refuse to go to the bathroom are putting themselves at risk of developing _____.

The correct answer is: (A) Incontinence.

The term 'incontinence' is used in reference to the inability to control urination or defecation. Some people develop incontinence because of an underlying medical problem, but as indicated in this question, consistently refusing to void one's bowels or bladder can also lead to the problem. Sometimes doctors may prescribe medication to alleviate incontinence, enhancing bladder function so it can be completely emptied at the appropriate time. There are also medications that doctors prescribe to tighten the muscles and reduce incidences of leakage. If urine leakage is occurring due to bladder position or an enlarged prostrate, the doctor could recommend surgery. There are also instances where people experience incontinence with no underlying ailment. Such instances include when a person is intoxicated or extremely anxious, when bathrooms are not readily available, during sudden coughing or sneezing or during uncontrollable laughter.

(46) Which of the following is part of the normal grieving process?

The correct answer is: (B) anticipatory grieving.

Anticipatory grief happens before a person has experienced real loss. If, for instance, a person has an ailing close relative and the patient's health condition continues to deteriorate, the person concerned is likely to begin experiencing anticipatory grief prior to the ill person's death. In short, if there are issues overwhelming you at a time of loss, the kind of grieving you experience can be referred to as inhibited grieving. Defining grieving can be complicated, especially in cases where someone has suffered several simultaneous losses.

(47) Which of the following is not permitted when a patient is on a clear liquid diet?

The correct answer is: (C) orange juice with pulp.

The fact that there is pulp in the juice disqualifies it from being clear liquid, which is what the doctor ordered. The other beverages are all acceptable clear liquids.

(48) The doctor orders twice daily ambulation of a client who has a Foley catheter. The CNA should _____ before starting to ambulate the client.

The correct answer is: (C) Ensure the bag is positioned below the level of the client's bladder.

A Foley catheter is a thin sterile tube that doctors insert into a patient's bladder to drain urine. It is often left in the patient's bladder for some time, and because of that it is also referred to as an 'indwelling catheter.' When you maintain the client's bag below the level of the bladder, you prevent bacteria from migrating upwards from within the bag to enter the bladder as a result of gravity.

(49) When is it necessary to restrain a patient?

The correct answer is: (A) Under orders from a physician.

It is important that a CNA wait for an order from the physician before putting a patient in restraints. If any member of staff puts a patient in restraints without an order from a physician, this is a case of battery.

(50) You have a patient who has just eaten a bagel and consumed a big glass of apple juice. What is the best way to record the patient's fluid intake?

The correct answer is: (C) 480 ml.

Within the field of medicine, the use of the term 'cc' has been replaced by 'ml.'

(51) There is a patient in the unit whom the doctor has put on airborne precautions because of suspicion of tuberculosis. The doctor has ordered that specimens of the patient's sputum be taken so he can then have them analyzed. What is the appropriate time of the day for the CNA to collect the specimens on a daily basis?

The correct answer is: (C) Early in the morning before the patient has done anything else.

The reason early morning is the best time to collect specimen sputum is that a patient's sputum is highly concentrated at this hour— more so than at any other time of day— and is therefore likely to yield the best results in terms of accuracy.

(52) If a CNA enters a patient's room and finds him masturbating, which of the following is the best action to take?

The correct answer is: (A) Instantly leave the patient's room to accord him privacy.

Since masturbation is a healthy way to express oneself sexually, the CNA should not do anything that can embarrass the patient. For that reason the most appropriate thing to do is quietly exit the room and keep away long enough to accord privacy to the patient.

(53) A CNA is dealing with a patient who is yelling, screaming and trying to bite her. What action should the CNA take?

The correct answer is: (B) Speak authoritatively but calmly to the patient.

When you speak calmly to a patient, even when your voice has authority, you are likely to be soothing and thereby reduce agitation. It is not necessary to use restraints on a patient who is experiencing confusion, especially when there is room to successfully placate him or her.

(54) A terminally ill client tells the CNA he has gotten into the habit of praying every night and believes God is going to forgive him. Which of the following stages of grief is the patient going through?

The correct answer is: (B) Bargaining.

When a patient begins praying to be forgiven when terminally ill, he or she is said to be in the bargaining stage of grief, which is normal in the grieving process.

(55) A CNA wants to help a patient who has been immobilized by disease to leave the bed and move to a chair. Which of the following is the best equipment for the CNA to use?

The correct answer is: (A) A transfer belt.

CNAs and other medical staff use transfer belts in order to safely carry a patient from one place to another as it enables the person helping the patient to maintain a better grip on the patient. In fact, using a transfer belt minimizes the risk of dropping the patient while moving him or her. A transfer belt not only provides safety for the patient but also for the CNA helping the patient move. Consequently, it is right to say a transfer belt helps prevent injury to both the patient and the CNA. It also ensures a patient remains comfortable during the move.

(56) A CNA is about to give a patient a bath just before bedtime. However, the CNA notices the patient has a Foley catheter in place, which means she needs to secure it to ensure there is no risk of it being pulled out when the patient is being bathed. Where should the CNA secure the catheter?

The correct answer is: (B) To the patient's thigh's lateral aspect.

Once the CNA secures the Foley catheter to the patient's thigh's lateral aspect, it is unlikely to be accidentally pulled out during the bath. Besides probably requiring the Foley catheter to be replaced, such accidental pulling of the catheter would cause the patient unnecessary pain.

(57) A patient who has just received terrible news that his wife has died is distraught as he tells the CNA he can't believe what he has just been told. He tells the CNA that he can't see how he can live without his wife. Which of the following is the best response from the CNA?

The correct answer is: (A) I know you are in real pain. I'll stay here and keep you company.

By giving this response, a CNA is echoing reality because the patient is in pain. The part of the response that indicates the CNA is prepared to keep the patient company is also important as part of the job entails comforting and providing empathy to mitigate the pain of loss.

(58) A CNA is helping a patient to bathe, and that patient has recently suffered a stroke on his right side. In order to enhance the patient's independence, the CNA should
_____.

The correct answer is: (C) Permit the patient to participate in his bathing as much as possible.

The best thing for a CNA to do in such a situation is to help the patient bathe even as he or she allows the patient to do what he can in the process. This way, though the patient may not do much bathing for himself at first, he is likely to improve and play a bigger role in his bathing as days go by. Such gradual progression is what often leads to full independence with time, where a patient who has had a one-sided stroke ends up being able to function properly without much help.

(59) A patient has burned his leg after accidentally pouring some hot soup on it. The skin is red and blistered. According to the CNA, this is a case of _____.

The correct answer is: (C) Partial thickness burn.

The look of a total thickness burn is both whitish and waxy, and a superficial burn (also known as a first-degree burn) involves blotchy skin and no blistering whatsoever. A partial thickness burn is also referred to as a second-degree burn, and it is worse than a superficial burn. Partial thickness burns penetrate the skin layers more deeply than a superficial burn, cause more pain and are more prone to infection. When a patient has a full thickness burn, it means both the epidermis and dermis, the two main skin layers, have been destroyed. It also means there is a chance the burn has gone deeper and reached other body structures that lie beneath the skin layers. When a patient has a full thickness burn, the sensory nerves are destroyed within the dermis. This means the patient can't feel any sensation if a pinprick test is done.

(60) The CNA notices a client has experienced no bowel movements for four days. Which procedure listed below would be most beneficial to the client?

The correct answer is: (C) An enema.

An enema helps to expel fecal matter from the patient's body before it can become impacted. The procedure entails liquid or gas being injected into a patient's rectum in order to expel the contents within it. Other times the procedure is carried out for the sake of introducing a given drug or to enable X-ray imaging.

# Test 2: Questions

(1) Since patients who have osteoarthritis can be put on bed rest for long durations, CNAs should be aware _____.

(A) Of the need to reduce stimulation while providing only passive motion

(B) Of the need to turn the patient at intervals of two hours while encouraging coughing and deep breathing

(C) Of the need to keep the client lying still and provide sufficient massage

(D) Of the need to encourage the patient to cough and take deep breaths while also limiting the intake of fluids


(2)   A patient has a leg in a cast and the nurse on duty instructs Mary, the CNA, to elevate the limb. If Mary _____, she will be elevating the patient's limb in the correct manner.

(A)   Puts the limb in the cast right below the patient's heart level

(B)   Puts the limb in the cast right above the patient's heart level

(C)   Puts the limb in the cast at the same level as the patient's heart

(D)   Puts the limb in the cast near the patient's body


(3)   The nurse on duty has received orders from the doctor that a particular patient should be restrained using a strait jacket. The nurse then delegates that task to the CNA, who is expected to know how to use such a type of restraint. Which of the following demonstrates an inappropriate use of a strait jacket?

(A)   Tying the safety knot within the straps of the restraint

(B)   Securing the strait jacket in a way that one is able to easily slide two fingers between the patient's skin and the restraint

(C)   Securing the restraints to the rails on the side of the bed

(D)   Securing the jacket's straps so they don't become tight when some force is applied them.

(4)    A nurse has inserted a Foley catheter into a patient with the aim of emptying the patient's bladder. Which of the following is an inappropriate procedure when a patient has an indwelling catheter?

(A)    Making sure the drainage bag is emptied every six to eight hours

(B)    Ensuring the tubing is positioned without dependent loops

(C)    Ensuring the drainage bag is attached to the lowest bedside rail and close to the patient's feet

(D)    Ensuring the drainage bag is placed below the level of the patient's bladder


(5)    Elderly patients often suffer stomachache and bloating. Which of the following should be avoided due to the propensity for bloating in elderly patients?

(A)    Cauliflower

(B)    Foods rich in protein

(C)    Prunes

(D)    Sodas


(6) The ideal water temperature for a Sitz bath that a CNA is administering is
_____.

(A) Temperature level ranging from $95°F - 110°F$

(B) Temperature level ranging from $65°F - 80°F$

(C) Temperature level ranging from $105°F - 120°F$

(D) Temperature level ranging from $80°F - 93°F$

(7)   A CNA has received instructions from the nurse that she must obtain a urinary specimen to test for sugar and ketones. This particular client has been diagnosed with diabetes mellitus. The CNA is expected to be aware that the specimen _____.

(A)   Should be obtained before the client has had breakfast

(B)   Should be obtained half an hour after eating as well as at bedtime

(C)   Should be obtained at bedtime

(D)   Should be obtained half an hour before eating and also at bedtime

(8)   A nurse asked the CNA to change a client's dressing that was not sterile. Which of the following is the correct procedure to follow?

(A)   The CNA should clean the client's wound then cover it well using a clean dressing and then carefully tape the bandage's edges

(B)   The CNA should tactfully refuse the assignment as CNAs' knowledge of wound dressing is limited

(C)   When cleaning the wound, the CNA should begin from the area of the skin away from the wound and follow longitudinal strokes while moving closer and closer to the wound

(D)   As the CNA changes the client's dressing, he or she should make a mental note of the color of the old dressing's drainage, its odor and amount, as well as its consistency

(9)   Which of the following is correct pertaining to ostomy care?

(A)   The patient concerned is able to defecate in a normal way

(B)   Ostomy care is carried out using a sterile technique

(C)   In order to change ostomy pouches, a physician must first issue orders

(D)   It is fine for patients to perform the procedure on their own once a qualified nurse has taught them

(10) A doctor has issued orders for a patient with Deep Vein Thrombosis (DVT) to wear elastic stockings. If the CNA _____, the action will be considered correct.

(A) Performs the required stocking application as the patient is seated on a chair

(B) Performs the required stocking application as the patient lies in bed

(C) Performs the required stocking application as the patient is seated on the bed with feet dangling

(D) Performs the required stocking application as the patient stands


(11) A CNA should understand that elastic stockings _____.

(A)   Prevent pressure sores

(B)   Prevent blood clots

(C)   Reduce swelling following an injury

(D)   Hold dressings in proper position


(12) A patient with COPD was admitted on the first floor of a facility a few days ago. In a bid to assist this patient, the CNA can _____.

(A) Make a decision on the most suitable device to utilize

(B) Turn on the oxygen

(C) Ensure the connecting tubing is secure and has no kinks

(D) Make a point of turning the oxygen either on or off as necessary

(13)  Once a CNA has applied an elastic bandage to a patient's right leg, it is crucial that she observe the leg for color and check its temperature _____.

(A) At intervals of two hours

(B) At intervals of a quarter of an hour

(C) In hourly intervals

(D) During every shift


(14)  Which of the following statements is correct pertaining to binders?

(A) A double T-binder is meant to be used exclusively for male patients

(B) Breast binders can be used to relieve breastfeeding women's discomfort

(C) In order to secure a straight abdominal binder, a CNA must assist a patient into a side-lying position, so as to be able to close the binder at the back with safety pins

(D) When straight abdominal binders are required, a client needs to be seated in a chair.


(15)  Often protective devices are used as treatment for pressure ulcers and skin breakdown. Which of the following is unlikely to be used for such treatment?

(A) A rubber sheet

(B) Flotation pads

(C) Trochanter rolls

(D) A bed cradle

(16) CNAs should monitor patients who need oxygen therapy so as to notice if they develop hypoxia. Some of the first signs of hypoxia are _____.

(A) Cyanosis as well as an increase in the patient's pulse rate

(B) Being able to breathe well only when seated

(C) Increase in a patient's temperature as well as decrease in respiration

(D) The patient being restless, dizzy and disoriented


(17) Jane, a CNA, finds that a patient who is asthmatic has developed dyspnea, and she knows that to relieve the patient he needs to be put in an orthopneic position. This position involves _____.

(A) Positioning the patient on a high backrest while hyperextending the patient's neck

(B) Putting the bedrest at a right angle

(C) Positioning the patient against a high backrest by making use of a pillow

(D) Positioning the patient in a sitting position as he or she leans over a table covered with a pillow


(18) Which of the following is an incorrect manner for a CNA to floss a patient's teeth?

(A) Holding the floss between the center fingers of either hand

(B) Gently moving the floss upwards and downwards in between the patient's teeth

(C) Using a fresh piece of floss for every tooth

(D) Flossing the back part of the farthest tooth and also on all sides—top, right and left as well as at the bottom of the mouth

(19)  In collecting a 24-hour urine specimen, the CNA should _____.

(A) Keep a 30 ml specimen from every voiding after recording the quantity voided, and this should be over a period of 24 hours

(B) Collect each sample in a different container over a period of 24 hours

(C) Record the timing and quantity of urine over a period of 24 hours

(D) Get rid of the first voiding, and then collect the entire volume of every voiding for 24 hours

(20)  Tom is a patient who has a hearing aid. He is deemed to be using the device properly when he wears it, turns it on and then adjusts it to _____.

(A) A level that has been prescribed

(B) A level that is therapeutic

(C) A level that is audible

(D) A level that has been preset

(21)  James is a patient who has just suffered a stroke, and all the signs he is manifesting relate to receptive aphasia. With regard to patients who have receptive aphasia, it is correct to say _____.

(A) They always speak with a loud voice

(B) They can easily understand spoken and written language

(C) They can't speak at all

(D) They don't have the capacity to speak well enough to express what they mean

(22) It's a CNA's responsibility to maintain an accurate record of I & O. In the case of a patient who is incontinent, which of the following is the best way to document a patient's output?

(A) There is no need to document the patient's output because it is difficult to measure

(B) Report to the nurse the moment the patient voids or defecates

(C) Make a point of reviewing the patient's intake, and then record the same amount of output on the I & O's output side

(D) Every time the patient wets the bed, record it on the I & O's output side


(23) Which of the following indicates fluid output requiring recording on a patient's I & O sheet?

(A) Urine as well as blood loss

(B) Urine

(C) Urine, blood loss and emesis as well as increased perspiration

(D) Urine and blood loss as well as increased perspiration


(24) Abdul is a client who is being given oxygen therapy through a face mask. Which of the following is contraindicated for Abdul?

(A) Engaging in talk with incoming visitors

(B) Using cotton bedsheets

(C) Consuming his own lunch

(D) Making use of an electric razor to shave

(25) Which of the following articles of clothing would be most helpful to a patient with osteoarthritis when it comes to performing everyday chores?

(A) Shoes that are properly tied in order to enhance stability

(B) Clothing that is buttoned, rubber grippers and slip-on shoes

(C) Clothing that is zippered

(D) Velcro clothing and rubber grippers as well as slip-on shoes


(26) Which of the following types of care does not pertain to patients fitted with pacemakers?

(A) Not permitted to work with a microwave

(B) Should make a point of avoiding magnetic wands used in airports

(C) Should be monitored in relation to the use of cellular phones

(D) Should not be near any electrical appliances


(27) Timothy's bowel movements have produced black stool with a tarry consistency. As a CNA, you should immediately _____.

(A) Ask the nurse to look at Timothy's stool

(B) Dispose of the black stool and then inform the nurse of what color Timothy's stool was

(C) Ask a fellow CNA if the black stool color is normal for Timothy

(D) Ask Timothy what he ate last

(28) In collecting specimens for medical use, certain rules should be followed. Which of the following is not such a rule?

(A) Accurately label the patient's specimen container

(B) Adhere to the regulations pertaining to medical asepsis

(C) Only collect the needed specimens when you can afford time

(D) Be careful to use the right container


(29) A CNA is expected to change bed linens for a patient who has a draining pressure ulcer. Which of the following should the CNA wear for protection before beginning the process of changing the patient's soiled bedsheets?

(A) A mask

(B) Shoe protectors

(C) Clean gloves

(D) Sterile gloves


(30) A patient has an indwelling urinary catheter. There is urine leaking out of a hole in the patient's collection bag. Because of that leakage, the CNA should _____.

(A) Disconnect the patient's drainage bag from the catheter and then replace it with an entirely new bag

(B) Place a towel beneath the bag to prevent urine from spilling onto the floor, as such an eventuality could make the client slip and probably fall

(C) Use some tape to seal the hole

(D) Report the leakage to the nurse immediately

(31) Which of the following is most suitable for urine collection?

(A) Have the patient start the urine stream from the toilet and then trap the urine midway in a sterile container

(B) Ensure you have cleaned the penis foreskin before collecting a urine sample from an uncircumcised man

(C) Have the patient void into the urinal and then pour the urine into the specimen container

(D) Ensure the patient voids into a clean container

(32) A CNA is performing penile hygiene on an unconscious patient. The CNA is carrying out the task correctly if he or she _____.

(A) Uses warm water and no soap

(B) Carries out the washing beginning at the shaft base and moves up towards the tip

(C) Thoroughly dries the entire penis

(D) Carefully retracts the patient's foreskin in the event that patient is uncircumcised.

(33) A CNA needs to take a patient's blood pressure within airborne isolation. Which of the following methods is best for preventing infection transmission to other patients through the use of equipment?

(A) Wearing gloves when using the equipment

(B) Using the equipment solely within airborne isolation

(C) Leaving the equipment in the room for the sole use of that initial patient

(D) Disposing of the equipment immediately following its use

(34) Which of the following is the best method for a CNA to apply an elastic bandage on a patient's arm for the purpose of preventing impairment of the circulation system?

(A) Applying great pressure each time the CNA turns the bandage

(B) Wrapping the bandage loosely around the patient's arm

(C) Beginning to apply the bandage from the upper part of the arm and working toward the lower part

(D) Applying the bandage while at the same time making a point of stretching it a bit


(35) Peter is a resident in a facility for elderly people and a CNA there has updated his I & O record. The record indicates intake as 180 ml of milk; 60 ml of juice; one serving of scrambled eggs; one slice of toast; one can of 240 ml as oral nutrition supplement and 50 ml of water to accompany medications taken two times in a day. The nurse administers medication at 9 a.m. and also at 9 p.m. What should the medical staff working the shift starting at 7 a.m. and ending at 3 p.m. consider to be the patient's intake?

(A) 550 ml

(B) 590 ml

(C) 580 ml

(D) 530 ml


(36) A CNA is about to put a patient who has an indwelling urinary catheter to bed when she notices there is tubing hanging beneath the patient's bed. She places the tubing on the patient's bed in the form of a loop while ensuring the patient does not lie on it. Which of the following indicates the rationale behind the CNA's actions?

(A) To facilitate urine collection within the tubing

(B) To inhibit drainage

(C) To facilitate drainage

(D) So that the patient can check whether the tubing has urine

(37) A client known as Irene has been put under suicide precautions. At a conference, the nursing staff discussed Irene's care plan. In order to ensure Irene's safety, the nurse can delegate certain tasks to the CNA. Such tasks include _____.

(A) Staying with the patient at all times

(B) Removing every object that is sharp or which has the capacity to cut

(C) Giving the patient a chance to express her feelings

(D) Not allowing the patient to leave her room


(38) A CNA instructs a patient who has Alzheimer's to brush his teeth. Instead of proceeding to brush his teeth, the patient exclaims, "Vanilla yogurt!" The best course of action for the CNA is to _____.

(A) Brush the patient's teeth for him

(B) Give the patient step-by-step instructions

(C) Focus on the patient's emotional reaction

(D) Provide the patient with clarification on what the instructions meant


(39) When a CNA identifies a patient with a history of attempted suicide, the CNA should _____.

(A) Invite a priest

(B) Report the information to the local police

(C) Counsel the patient

(D) Report the information immediately to the nurse

(40) A man who was formerly a drug addict is now 33 years of age and is paralyzed from the waist downwards. No family members came to visit him during the time he was hospitalized, but there was talk that he had two teenage sons. As a CNA, how can you help the patient meet his relationship needs and those needs associated with his role as a family person?

(A) Spend reasonable time with the patient after working hours

(B) Get some people to send the patient anonymous get well cards

(C) Give him some alone time to meditate

(D) Give him writing materials so that he can write to his two sons


(41)  It is the right of patients and their families to benefit from care _____.

(A) That medical research has proved to be appropriate

(B) That the team of medical professionals has found to be appropriate

(C) That is culturally suitable for them

(D) That is advanced in terms of technology and reasonably priced.


(42)  There are certain things medical staff need to do at different stages of a patient's treatment. In the case of a patient who is close to death, the CNA should _____.

(A) Help the patient have peaceful final days

(B) Motivate the patient to reach a peaceful death

(C) Encourage the patient to become as independent as possible

(D) Help the patient to carry out normal duties on a day-to-day basis

(43) Sometimes patients who have a terminal disease refuse to believe they are faced with imminent loss, and they feign cheerfulness. This stage of the grieving process is referred to as _____.

(A) Depression

(B) Acceptance

(C) Denial

(D) Bargaining


(44) In a bid to respect a patient's values including those of a cultural nature, you may wish to include foods commonly valued in the patient's community. If you want to show cultural sensitivity when caring for a Hispanic patient, you might incorporate _____ in the patient's meals.

(A) Potatoes as well as red meat

(B) Beans as well as tortillas

(C) Rice and vegetables

(D) Cheese and varieties of olive oil


(45) A CNA wants to interview a patient who is 93 years of age. Which of the following is the most suitable interviewing technique?

(A) Using pictures to reinforce what the CNA says in words

(B) Making sure to enunciate words slowly

(C) Making sure to vary voice intonations while speaking

(D) Speaking in a low-pitched voice

(46) A 68-year-old woman has been diagnosed with colon cancer. The woman has daughters with the power of attorney, and they have demanded that their mother not be told of her diagnosis. After the daughters have left, the woman asks the CNA about her illness and diagnosis. Which of the following is the best answer for the CNA to give?

(A) I'm sorry, you should direct that question to the doctor and not me

(B) In my view you are in pretty good shape and don't need to worry

(C) I promise to check out what is happening and get back to you. For now though, I have no information

(D) Sorry, I have no information pertaining to your illness


(47) A patient who has been in a long-term health care facility for a year tells the CNA, "I can't even talk with you considering how depressed I am. Just forget about me." Which of the following is the most appropriate response?

(A) I'll stay right here in the room with you for a while

(B) Just wait here. I'll return in an hour's time

(C) Just reach out to me when you're in the mood for talking

(D) Why do you think you're depressed?


(48) Suppose a patient you are taking care of says to you, "I feel worthless. I should not even be alive." Which of the following is the most appropriate response?

(A) That's a lie

(B) I'll help you get over these negative feelings

(C) What is it that gives you that feeling of worthlessness?

(D) Stop saying you should not be alive since the truth is that you are worthy of living.

(49) A hearing impaired patient is taken to the hospital and the unit where he is admitted is very busy. People with hearing impairments can suffer sensory overload. Which of the following interventions is appropriate to prevent this from happening?

(A) Ensure there is an overhead light on where the patient is

(B) Allow the patient's family members to remain with him

(C) Ensure that there is a TV or radio on near the patient's location at all times

(D) Make a point of conversing with the patient from his bedside


(50) Which of the following is accurate pertaining to patients' charts?

(A) Patients' charts are the property of the hospital and nobody else should have access to them even on request other than the doctor who is in charge of the patient

(B) Patients' charts are the property of the government because they are considered legal documents

(C) Patients' charts are the property of the respective patients and the CNA should give them to the patients on request

(D) Patients' charts are the property of the doctor who is in charge of the patients and under no circumstances should they be given to the hospital administrator


(51) Jane, a CNA, has been charged with taking the vitals of a number of residents in a long-term facility. She carries out the task but fails to take the vitals of one of the residents. The nurse who oversees the CNA's work notices there is some information missing, and she asks the CNA about it. The CNA admits her error. The fact that she owned up exemplifies _____.

(A) Respectability

(B) Flexibility

(C) Accountability

(D) Dependability

(52) Susan used to work as a CNA in a long-term facility, but she left two years ago to care for her newborn baby. For the last two years she has been a full-time mother, but now she has opted to resume work as a CNA to help pay increasing bills. What requirements will Susan have to fulfill in order to qualify to resume work as a CNA?

(A) Take a refresher course for CNAs

(B) Take an evaluation test for competency

(C) Present a formal letter to the relevant board showing intent to resume work as CNA

(D) Retrain as a CNA and then go through the competency evaluation again

(53) It is a very busy Monday for the staff on your ward. The duty nurse hands you Terramycin ointment in its normal tube as she continues to prepare other medications for patients from the usual medication tray. She instructs you to apply that ointment to the eyes of a particular patient. What is the most appropriate response to her instruction?

(A) Ask her to watch as you apply the ointment

(B) Ask that she demonstrate how you apply the appointment

(C) Politely say that you are not authorized as a CNA to apply the ointment

(D) Administer the ointment to the patient as per her instructions

(54) A nurse who serves as a CNA's supervisor emphasizes the need for communication among members of the medical staff. The importance of this, according to the nurse, is to ensure care is given to individual patients in a manner that is coordinated and also effective. Communication by the CNA includes every one of the suggestions listed below apart from one. Which one is the exception?

(A) Being not only brief but also concise

(B) Providing facts and being specific

(C) Using terms that have several meanings

(D) Presenting information in a logical manner and also in sequence

(55) A CNA receives a call while on duty only to realize the caller wants to speak to someone in a different medical unit. What is the best response?

(A) The CNA should tell the caller to hold for the operator and then resume the tasks she was carrying out before the call came in

(B) The CNA should alert the nurse about the call so the nurse herself can redirect it to the right unit

(C) The CNA should promise to redirect the call to the correct unit but also provide the person with the correct number in case the call is disconnected or the other unit's line is busy

(D) The CNA should ask the caller the number he or she is trying to reach.


(56) You are working as a CNA in a long-term facility, and as you give one of the clients a bed bath a call comes in over the intercom. The unit secretary wants to alert the unit of an emergency phone call just coming in. The most suitable action for you to take is

_____.

(A) Hurry from the room from where you are giving the client a bath and pick up the call

(B) Ignore the call and finish bathing the client first

(C) Cover the client and put the call light close to him or her, then respond to the call

(D) Leave the door to the client's room open to facilitate monitoring, then go answer the emergency call

(57)  In the facility where you are working as a CNA, you have received a new client. In order to facilitate proper care, you need some medical history pertaining to the client. This includes the nature of nursing support the client was receiving previously and what therapeutic management the client received before, if any.

To get that information, you need to read the _____.

(A) Notes on the client's progress

(B) Flow sheet

(C) Nursing discharge summary

(D) Kardex


(58)  It's time for the nursing round and as the team moves from one room to another they find a patient lying flat on the floor. Something must be entered in the patient's medical record. Which of the following is it most likely the CNA will record pertaining to the incident?

(A) If there was a bed alarm available the patient would likely not have fallen

(B) There is a chance the patient tried to climb over the bed rails and ended up falling

(C) The patient was restless the entire evening and ended up attempting to move out of bed

(D) On entering the patient's room, the patient was discovered lying flat on the floor

(59) Patients' medical records are held at the facility in confidentiality. However, if staff members are not careful they can make mistakes that can compromise such confidentiality. Given that patients' records are computerized, what can put their confidentiality at risk?

(A) Sharing personal passwords with other members of staff so they can access the computer when they can't remember their own passwords

(B) Preventing someone unknown to you but who tells you he is a member of staff from reading medical records

(C) Logging off and signing off from all computers before you leave the terminal

(D) Changing your computer passwords periodically


(60) A registered nurse is taking you around for orientation in a facility where you are newly employed as a CNA. She informs you that it is usual for patients from diverse cultures to be admitted to the facility, and some of them converse in languages other than English. What is the appropriate thing to do when faced with such patients?

(A) Ensure you always speak to them loudly and slowly

(B) Ensure you always speak to the patient when family members are around because that increases the chance of what you are saying being understood

(C) Ensure you stand near the patient as you speak slowly

(D) Use an interpreter whenever you need to communicate with the patient

# Test 2: Answers & Explanations

(1) Since patients who have osteoarthritis can be put on bed rest for long durations, CNAs should be aware _____.

The correct answer is: (B) Of the need to turn the patient at intervals of two hours while encouraging coughing and deep breathing.

Bedridden patients should be turned every two hours and must be encouraged to cough and take deep breaths so as to prevent possible complications of pneumonia or pressure ulcers. Such patients also need to be fed a nutritious diet. The massage suggested in some answer options is fine for reduction of pain, but it is not helpful to keep the patient constantly still.

ROM exercises are helpful for the patient, but such motion does not have to be just passive; even active motion is helpful. The exercises are described as 'active' if the patient can do them on his own, and they are described as passive when the patient can only make the movements with the assistance of equipment or someone else such as a therapist or a CNA. It is also helpful to keep the patient well hydrated by providing sufficient fluids, which means the answer option suggesting that fluids be limited is wrong.

(2)   A patient has a leg in a cast and the nurse on duty instructs Mary, the CNA, to elevate the limb. If Mary _____, she will be elevating the patient's limb in the correct manner.

The correct answer is: (B) Puts the limb in the cast right above the patient's heart level.

The reason it is recommended that a patient's limb be placed right above the level of his heart when in a cast is to bring down any swelling. In order for the limb to remain in that position, the CNA should place pillows right below it for support. If the CNA places the limb either at the same level with the patient's heart or below the heart level, the swelling will not lessen. Placing the limb close to the patient's body is erroneous because in order to elevate the limb to the required level, the CNA might have to extend it somewhat away from the patient's body.

(3)   The nurse on duty has received orders from the doctor that a particular patient should be restrained using a strait jacket. The nurse then delegates that task to the CNA, who is expected to know how to use such a type of restraint. Which of the following demonstrates an inappropriate use of a strait jacket?

The correct answer is: (C) Securing the restraints to the rails on the side of the bed

The reason this is an inappropriate action to take is that if the side rail gets released the patient could be accidentally injured. The right place to secure the restraint straps is the frame of the bed and not the side rails. Tying the safety knot within the straps of the restraint is appropriate. In fact, either a safety knot or a half bow is recommended for use during an application of a restraint owing to the fact that it does not become tight when there is force applied on it or against it. This safety knot is also suitable for use because it allows for fast and easy removal of the jacket during an emergency. Securing the jacket's restraints in a way that one is able to easily slide two fingers between the patient's skin and that restraint is appropriate.


(4)   A nurse has inserted a Foley catheter into a patient with the aim of emptying the patient's bladder. Which of the following is an inappropriate procedure when a patient has an indwelling catheter?

The correct answer is: (C) Ensuring the drainage bag is attached to the lowest bedside rail and close to the patient's feet.

Normally the drainage bag is positioned in a manner that leaves it hanging from a chair or bed frame, or a patient's wheelchair. At no time should the drainage bag ever be left touching the floor. Nevertheless, positioning the drainage bag below the patient's bladder is the right thing to do. The reason the bag should never be positioned above the level of the patient's bladder is that in that position there is a chance of the urine flowing back into the patient's bladder, potentially causing an infection. For this reason, option (C) that indicates the drainage bag should be placed closest to the patient's feet as it is attached to the side rail is incorrect. Positioning a patient's drainage bag in this manner would be inappropriate, and moreover, it would mean whenever the rail gets raised the bag will move above the level of the patient's bladder. If the patient is walking, the drainage bag should always be below the level of the bladder.

It is correct to say the drainage bag should be emptied every six to eight hours in order to avoid microbe proliferation and infection. The action in option (B) is appropriate because that ensures there is no risk of urine stasis within the tubes, because that might enhance the chances of urine flowing backwards into the patient's bladder.

(5)   Elderly patients often suffer stomachache and bloating. Which of the following should be avoided due to the propensity for bloating in elderly patients?

The correct answer is: (A) Cauliflower.

Cauliflower is known to cause bloating because it causes gas to form. Food items that similarly form gas in the stomach include cabbage and cucumber, radishes and beans. There are numerous foods that can cause gas including lentils and carbohydrates like pasta and bread, if eaten in large quantities. For anyone lactose intolerant, whether elderly or not, consuming any kind of dairy products can lead to bloating.


(6)   The ideal water temperature for a Sitz bath that a CNA is administering is
_____.

The correct answer is: (A) Temperature level ranging from $95°F - 110°F$.

The ideal temperature of the bathwater falls in between $95°F$ and goes all the way up to $110°F$, because within this range of temperatures the client is likely to relax and be comfortable. Within this range, temperatures are neither too hot nor too cold for the client. If the water temperature falls below $95°F$, it begins to lose its effectiveness in relaxing the client, and at some level it even begins to cause the client's muscles to tighten. If this happens it means the purpose of the Sitz bath, which is to relax the muscles, is being negated. In fact, a Sitz bath at the right range of temperatures not only relaxes but also relieves muscle spasms and hastens the healing process, especially after perianal surgery. A good Sitz bath has several other benefits to the client, including relieving congestion and hastening the process of suppuration for patients with related health issues.

(7)    A CNA has received instructions from the nurse that she must obtain a urinary specimen to test for sugar and ketones. This particular client has been diagnosed with diabetes mellitus. The CNA is expected to be aware that the specimen _____.

The correct answer is: (D) Should be obtained half an hour before eating and also at bedtime.

In cases of diabetes, sugar has been known to appear in a person's urine; what is referred to as glucosuria or even glycosuria. The person being tested may also have acetones in the urine if diabetic, which are essentially ketones or ketone bodies. To determine whether a patient has sugar or ketones in his or her urine, tests are carried out four times a day—half an hour before eating each meal and then again at bedtime.

For best results from these particular tests, the specimens should be double-voided. Double-voided specimens are collected twice at the same time, the first time the normal way and the second time after waiting in the urinating position for 20 to 30 seconds for more urine.

(8)    A nurse asked the CNA to change a client's dressing that was not sterile. Which of the following is the correct procedure to follow?

The correct answer is: (D) As the CNA changes the client's dressing, he or she should make a mental note of the color of the old dressing's drainage, its odor and amount, as well as its consistency.

The reason all the options apart from option (D) are incorrect is that, while it is fine to tape a bandage securely into place, its edges should be left free. That makes option (A) incorrect. As for refusing the task, as suggested in option (B), it is wrong as all CNAs should anticipate doing wound dressings that don't call for sterile techniques. It is considered their duty just as application of medication to clients' wounds is one of the many tasks assigned to them. Option (C) is incorrect as wounds are supposed to be cleaned in circular movements and not in longitudinal strokes. Also, the cleaning should be done starting from the part considered the cleanest to the one considered the dirtiest. In this case, the wound is considered the cleanest and the further away you move from the wound the dirtier it is considered to be.

(9)    Which of the following is correct pertaining to ostomy care?

The correct answer is: (D) It is fine for patients to perform the procedure on their own once a qualified nurse has taught them.

Ostomy care should be done as per the rules pertaining to cleanliness; aseptically. A CNA does not need any orders from a physician in order to change a patient's ostomy pouch. There are specific times when the pouch should be changed, including when the pouch has filled up or if the seal has broken. When a patient has an ostomy, it is expected that the nature of his or her bowel movement will change. There is an appliance through which the patient's fecal material is collected, and this appliance is held above the patient's stoma—the hollow passage into the gut—using paste or a unique adhesive.

(10)   A doctor has issued orders for a patient with Deep Vein Thrombosis (DVT) to wear elastic stockings. If the CNA _____, the action will be considered correct.

The correct answer is: (B) Performs the required stocking application as the patient lies in bed.

The normal way of going about stocking application when a patient has DVT is to do it before it becomes necessary for the patient to leave his or her bed. The CNA should avoid applying the stockings while the patient is in a sitting or standing position because those positions are known to exacerbate the swelling of the legs. When patients with DVT don't have elastic stockings on, they should remain lying on their beds so that the legs don't swell; or if their legs are swollen already, the position will ensure the swelling doesn't become more serious.

(11)   A CNA should understand that elastic stockings _____.

The correct answer is: (B) Prevent blood clots.

Elastic stockings are good at preventing blood clots by exerting pressure and enhancing blood circulation through the veins and into the heart. Generally elastic stockings are used in providing compression therapy to patients with venous pressure and leg aches. They are also known to prevent venous stasis while also preventing impairment of a person's venous walls. Venous stasis is a state that raises a person's risk factor for clot formation within the blood veins.

(12)  There is a patient with COPD who was admitted on the first floor of the facility a few days ago. In a bid to assist this patient, the CNA can _____.

The correct answer is: (C) Ensure the connecting tubing is secure and has no kinks.

It is the CNA's responsibility to ensure the patient's connecting tubing has no kinks, and that it is secured well in place. Every other responsibility mentioned on the list of answer options, including making a decision on the most appropriate device to use, turning on the oxygen and turning the oxygen on or off as necessary, falls under the role of the physician. This basically means that once the physician has chosen a suitable device for the patient and started the flow of oxygen, the CNA's job is to ensure the connecting tubing is not interfered with in any way.


(13)  Once a CNA has applied an elastic bandage to a patient's right leg, it is crucial that she observe the leg for color and check its temperature _____.

The correct answer is: (C) In hourly intervals.

As the CNA applies the elastic bandage, it is important that she leave the patient's toes or fingers exposed, because that is how she will be able to check blood circulation. She should check the extremities for both color and temperature each hour. If the CNA finds that the patient is having a tingling sensation, feeling pain, is itching or feeling numb, she should inform the nurse immediately. There are some basics that CNAs should observe to ensure a patient is both safe and comfortable. Among these is ensuring a bandage has not been fixed so tightly that it impedes blood flow. It is also recommended that a bandage be removed a minimum of two times a day for a few minutes. In some cases the doctor or nurse may order the bandage to be removed at bedtime.

(14)  Which of the following statements is correct pertaining to binders?

(E) The correct answer is: (A) A double T-binder is meant to be used exclusively for male patients.

T-binders are used in securing dressings in position following rectal and perianal surgeries. Whereas medical staff is meant to use the double T-binder on men, they are supposed to use single T-binders on women. When the purpose is to support breasts following surgery, breast binders should be used. Therefore, the suggestion that breast binders are used by breastfeeding women is erroneous. For the straight abdominal binders, the patient needs to be in a supine position. As such, the option suggesting the patient should be seated in a chair is wrong. While the patient is in the supine position, the binder is secured into position at the front side of the patient's body by use of safety pins, zippers, Velcro, hooks or other closures. While the top part of the binder is level with the patient's waist, its lower part lies over the patient's hips.


(15)  Often protective devices are used as treatment for pressure ulcers and skin breakdown. Which of the following is unlikely to be used for such treatment?

The correct answer is: (A) A rubber sheet.

A rubber sheet is usually used to protect the patient from soiled linen and excessive drainage. Such foul conditions can lead to the patient developing ulcers or having skin breakdown, not only because of the moisture but also owing to the friction occasioned on the skin. As for trochanter rolls, their role is not to prevent pressure ulcers or breakdown of skin. They are actually used in preventing legs and hips from turning in an outward direction even as they assist in positioning a patient properly. A bed cradle is meant to be put on a patient's bed some distance above the patient, so that when the top bed linen is spread over it there is no pressure exerted on the patient's legs or feet.

(16)  CNAs should monitor patients who need oxygen therapy so as to notice if they develop hypoxia. Some of the first signs of hypoxia are _____.

The correct answer is: (D) The patient being restless, dizzy and disoriented.

The term 'hypoxia' is used in reference to the life-threatening condition where cells of the body do not have sufficient oxygen. Among the earliest signs of hypoxia are restlessness, dizziness and disorientation. Option (C) is outright wrong as hypoxia actually causes a person's rate of respiration to increase and not decrease. At the same time, hypoxia is not known to cause a rise in temperature. As for option (A), it is incorrect because although cyanosis is a sign of hypoxia, it surfaces late and not early.

(17)  Jane, a CNA, finds that a patient who is asthmatic has developed dyspnea, and she knows that to relieve the patient he needs to be put in an orthopneic position. This position involves _____.

The correct answer is: (D) Positioning the patient in a sitting position as he or she leans over a table covered with a pillow.

Whenever patients have difficulty breathing, they prefer to sit upright, but leaning over a table makes breathing easier. This is the position referred to as the orthopneic position. Place a pillow on the table for the patient's comfort.

(18)  Which of the following is an incorrect manner for a CNA to floss a patient's teeth?

The correct answer is: (C) Using a fresh piece of floss for every tooth.

It is unnecessary to use a fresh piece of floss for each tooth. To clean the entire range of teeth for the patient, the CNA just needs an 18-inch-long piece of floss. The best procedure is to shift to a new section of the piece of floss every two teeth. All the other options are correct procedures for flossing a patient's teeth.

(19)  In collecting a 24-hour urine specimen, the CNA should _____.

The correct answer is: (D) Get rid of the first voiding, and then collect the entire volume of every voiding for 24 hours.

What is described as a 24-hour urine specimen is all the urine collected from the patient over a span of 24 hours, and that is normally beginning from 7 a.m. of one day up to 7 a.m. of the next day. It is crucial that as a CNA you ask the patient to void first, and then get rid of that urine. This is because the urine just voided has been in the patient's bladder for an uncertain period of time. In short, the urine test should begin with an empty bladder. After that you need to retain all the urine that the patient voids in one bottle for a continuous 24-hour period. As for recording the amount of urine the patient voids every time and the exact time that amount was voided, it's not essential.


(20)  Tom is a patient who has a hearing aid. He is deemed to be using the device properly when he wears it, turns it on and then adjusts it to _____.

The correct answer is: (C) A level that is audible

A hearing device is meant to be set to a volume level that is audible to the patient. A hearing aid helps the patient hear better in both quiet and noisy environments. Hearing aids are important medical devices for people with hearing problems. Another term for loss of hearing is hearing impairment, which is sometimes partial and other times total. People with total hearing impairment who are unable to hear anything at all can be said to be deaf. Causes of hearing impairment are sometimes genetic and other times of a non-genetic nature. Those of a non-genetic nature include infection, ear trauma, complications at birth, advanced age, being exposed to immense noise, toxins and some medications.


(21)  James is a patient who has just suffered a stroke, and all the signs he is manifesting relate to receptive aphasia. With regard to patients who have receptive aphasia, it is correct to say _____.

The correct answer is (D) They don't have the capacity to speak well enough to express what they mean. The term 'aphasia' is used in reference to language impairment, which affects speech production or speech comprehension. It also affects a person's reading or writing capacity. Aphasia is caused by an injury to a person's brain mostly through stroke, and it is more prevalent in elderly people. Receptive aphasia is also referred to as Wernicke's aphasia. It is also referred to as 'sensory aphasia' or 'posterior aphasia.' Posterior aphasia is known for causing difficulty in understanding language, whether spoken or written.

(22)  It is the responsibility of a CNA to maintain an accurate record of I & O. In the case of a patient who is incontinent, which of the following is the best way to document a patient's output?

The correct answer is: (D) Every time the patient wets the bed, record it on the I & O sheet's output side.

Every time the patient wets the bed, the CNA needs to record it on the I & O sheet's output side. It is clear in such circumstances the CNA has no way of determining the quantity of urine the patient has voided, and once the patient has wet the bed it becomes evident his or her kidneys are functioning.

(23)  Which of the following indicate fluid output requiring recording on a patient's I & O sheet?

The correct answer is: (C) Urine, blood loss and emesis as well as increased perspiration.

When the term 'fluid output' is used in the medical field, it means the totality of all the fluids coming out of a person's body. The largest proportion of the fluid output is in the form of urine. This fluid output is also inclusive of vomitus, which is what is also referred to as emesis. It also includes any fluids being discharged from wounds, any blood loss or any excessive perspiration. This means it is incumbent upon the CNA to measure the fluid amount whenever the patient visits the urinal, makes use of the emesis basin or uses the bedpan. As for perspiration or discharge from a wound, the CNA should point out the exact thing that became wet and its degree of wetness. It is also important to indicate how big the wet part is, and also the time the wetness occurred.

(24) Abdul is a client who is being given oxygen therapy through a face mask. Which of the following is contraindicated for Abdul?

The correct answer is: (D) Making use of an electric razor to shave.

It is important for a patient receiving oxygen therapy to have safety measures implemented to prevent an explosion. For safety reasons, using an electric razor is not permitted as long as there is oxygen running. Likewise, a hair dryer should not be used in such circumstances. It is not even permissible to comb a patient's hair in proximity to an oxygen tank as a static spark could trigger an explosion. It's fine for the patient to remove the face mask when eating or talking with visitors. As for use of bed linen made of cotton, it is highly recommended because it reduces the chances of igniting static electricity.

(25) Which of the following articles of clothing would be most helpful to a patient with osteoarthritis when it comes to performing everyday chores?

The correct answer is: (D) Velcro clothing and rubber grippers as well as slip-on shoes

Velcro clothing, rubber grippers and slip-on shoes help patients to get dressed by allowing them to get a good grip on objects. It is important to note that items like buttons, ties and zippers are likely to be difficult for patients with osteoarthritis to handle.

(26) Which of the following types of care does not pertain to patients fitted with pacemakers?

The correct answer is: (D) Should not be near any electrical appliances.

The reason option (D) is the correct answer is that it is the option that is not applicable to a patient with a pacemaker. In actual fact, there is nothing to prevent a patient with a pacemaker from using an electrical appliance. Most common electrical gadgets within a home will not affect a person's pacemaker. Televisions and toasters, electric knives and blankets, microwaves, fitness trackers and heart-rate monitors are all safe for patients with pacemakers to use. As for magnetic wands that are installed in airports for security purposes, patients with pacemakers should avoid them. In some instances, patients who use pacemakers are uncomfortable when they are around cell phones or lawn mowers.

(27) Timothy's bowel movements have produced black stool with a tarry consistency. As a CNA, you should immediately _____.

The correct answer is: (A) Ask the nurse to look at Timothy's stool.

The CNA should always make a point of reporting any stool that appears abnormal to the nurse. It is important that the CNA and the nurse observe the stool very carefully in terms of its color, quantity, odor, size, consistency and shape. Other important factors that require monitoring include the frequency with which the patient defecates and also the complaints the patient raises regarding pain.

(28) In collecting specimens for medical use, certain rules should be followed. Which of the following is not such a rule?

The correct answer is: (C) Only collect the needed specimens when you can afford time.

It is not the norm to have CNAs collect specimens at their own leisure or convenience and for that reason option (C) is the correct answer. The reason for collecting specimens is for detecting and treating disease. It is the doctor who decides and orders the specimen that needs collection and what tests need to be carried out.

(29) A CNA is expected to change bed linens for a patient who has a draining pressure ulcer. Which of the following should the CNA wear for protection before beginning the process of changing the patient's soiled bedsheets?

The correct answer is: (C) Clean gloves.

Clean gloves serve to protect the CNA's hands and wrists from any microorganisms in the soiled linen. The reason the option with sterile gloves is incorrect is that you are supposed to use these when the intention is to avoid personally contaminating something or a sterile area. A mask is used for the protection of the wearer as well as the patient from large particles of aerosols and droplet nuclei. As for shoe protectors, they are used in preventing the transmission of microorganisms from one room's floor to another.

(30) A patient has an indwelling urinary catheter. There is urine leaking out of a hole in the patient's collection bag. Because of that leakage, the CNA should _____.

The correct answer is: (D) Report the leakage to the nurse immediately.

The system being used by the patient can no longer be considered a closed one owing to the hole where urine is leaking from the collection bag, so there is a probability bacteria may have entered the system. For this reason the CNA should immediately report the leakage to the nurse with a view to having the catheter replaced with a new one via the sterile technique. It would not be helpful to place a towel beneath the bag in order to avoid leakage, and the same applies to taping the hole. Both these actions would still leave the system with an opening through which bacteria could enter. Although a change of catheter is likely to happen after the matter is reported to the nurse, the CNA can't personally change the catheter as that task does not fall under a CNA's duties.

(31) Which of the following is most suitable for urine collection?

The correct answer is: (A) Have the patient start the urine stream from the toilet and then you must trap the urine midway, putting it into a sterile container.

Catching the patient's urine midway is recommended as it reduces the chances of contaminating the specimen by microorganisms entering via the meatus or opening. The suggestion that voiding be done in the urinal is not suitable as the urinal is not sterile. Hence it cannot be guaranteed that a specimen collected from the urinal will be free of contamination. The option to clean an uncircumcised man's foreskin is erroneous as normally the recommendation in such a case is to retract the foreskin before cleaning the man's glans. The reason for this cleaning is to avoid possible contamination of the urine specimen. There are times when voiding is directed into a container that is clean, but this is done when the specimen being collected is just a random sample. However, when what is wanted is a clean-catch sample specifically for carrying out a urine culture, this method is not recommended.

(32) A CNA is performing penile hygiene on an unconscious patient. The CNA is carrying out the task correctly if he or she _____.

The correct answer is: (C) Thoroughly dries the entire penis.

It is essential to ensure the entire penis is well dried so that the penis is not macerated. When cleaning the penis, it is preferable to wash it starting at the tip and working down to the base in order to lessen the risk of introducing microorganisms into the patient's meatus. For effective cleaning the use of soap is recommended followed by proper rinsing. Secretions accumulated beneath the patient's foreskin also need to be removed, because they can cause inflammation. These secretions are also linked to penile cancer. It is also important to retract the foreskin of a man who is not circumcised before cleaning the penis, and then to replace it in order to avoid capistration or what is also referred to as paraphimosis. Paraphimosis is the condition where a man's penis fails to retract, mostly because of having been extended for a long time period, leading to swelling. The swelling of the penis then makes its sheath extra tight and that makes it difficult for the penis to retract.


(33) Which of the following methods is best for preventing infection transmission to other patients through the use of equipment?

The correct answer is: (C) Leaving the equipment in the room for the sole use of that initial patient.

It is appropriate to leave the equipment in the room you used it with your first patient to ensure the equipment is not contaminated by organisms on inanimate objects. Whereas disposing of equipment immediately following its use can effectively prevent organism transmission, the method is not at all cost-effective and is therefore not preferable. As for wearing gloves, it is great for the protection of the CNA but does not protect patients from transmitted organisms. In fact, the use of equipment previously used by other patients is a sure way of increasing the chances of spreading organisms of an infectious nature among patients.

(34) Which of the following is the best method for a CNA to apply an elastic bandage on a patient's arm for the purpose of preventing impairment of the circulation system?

The correct answer is: (D) Applying the bandage while at the same time making a point of stretching it a bit.

The reason it is important to stretch the elastic bandage a bit is to maintain uniformity in the tension of the bandage. It is inappropriate to apply the elastic bandage in a loose manner as that will not be effective in securing the bandage on the patient's arm. Applying great pressure to the bandage will impair the patient's blood circulation, and that fact makes option (A) inappropriate. Option (C) is also inappropriate as applying the elastic bandage beginning from the upper part of the arm is tantamount to applying the bandage unevenly. That is why, for example, application of elastic stockings is done distal to proximal for enhancement of venous return.

(35) Peter is a resident in a facility for elderly people and a CNA there has updated his I & O record. The record indicates intake as 180 ml of milk; 60 ml of juice; one serving of scrambled eggs; one slice of toast; one can of 240 ml as oral nutrition supplement and 50 ml of water to accompany medications taken two times in a day. The nurse administers medication at 9 a.m. and also at 9 p.m. What should the medical staff working the shift starting at 7 a.m. and ending at 3 p.m. consider to be the patient's intake?

The correct answer is: (D) 530 ml.

All you need to do to get the total intake by the patient is add all the fluids together: 180 ml + 60 ml +240 ml + 50 ml = 530 ml

(36) A CNA is about to put a patient who has an indwelling urinary catheter to bed when she notices there is tubing hanging beneath the patient's bed. She places the tubing on the patient's bed in the form of a loop while ensuring the patient does not lie on it. Which of the following indicates the rationale behind the CNA's actions?

The correct answer is: (C) To facilitate drainage.

It is not appropriate to let catheter tubing end up developing dependent loops or kinks, as such a development can inhibit good drainage by forcing urine to move against gravitational force in the process of being emptied into the drainage bag. The suggestion that urine could be facilitated to collect within the tubing is completely wrong because if that happens the risk of infection to the patient will be heightened. Option (D) is also wrong because it is not the responsibility of the patient to check whether the tubing has urine. That is the work of the nursing staff.

(37) A client known as Irene has been put under suicide precautions. At a conference, the nursing staff discussed Irene's care plan. In order to ensure Irene's safety, the nurse can delegate certain tasks to the CNA. Such tasks include _____.

The correct answer is: (A) Staying with the patient at all times.

Any patient who is under suicide precaution requires constant monitoring by a member of staff. This means there should always be a member of the nursing staff keeping the patient within sight, preferably within a distance of two to three feet of the patient no matter what activity the patient is engaged in, inclusive of the patient's visits to the bathroom. As for not allowing the patient to leave her room and removing every object that is sharp or has the capacity to cut; that is all part of maintaining a secure environment. Although it is good to give the patient a chance to vent, that should only happen after a patient's safety has been assured.

(38) A CNA instructs a patient who has Alzheimer's to brush his teeth. Instead of proceeding to brush his teeth, the patient exclaims, "Vanilla yogurt!" The best course of action for the CNA is to _____.

The correct answer is: (B) Give the patient step-by-step instructions.

It is clear the patient has a problem recognizing or naming objects, which is referred to as 'agnosia.' Such a patient needs to be given instructions one step at a time. It is not necessary to use any implements to guide the patient. It is sufficient to try and connect with the patient verbally.

(39) When a CNA identifies a patient with a history of attempted suicide, the CNA should _____.

The correct answer is: (D) Report the information immediately to the nurse.

By reporting the information immediately to the nurse, the CNA is ensuring the patient's safety. With this information, the nurse can refer the patient to an appropriate health care provider so that a proper assessment of the patient can be done along with planning for suitable care. Other tasks such as inviting a priest, reporting to the local police or giving counsel are not part of your duties as a CNA.

(40) A man who was formerly a drug addict is now 33 years of age and is paralyzed from the waist downwards. No family members came to visit him during the time he was hospitalized, but there was talk that he had two teenage sons. As a CNA, how can you help the patient meet his relationship needs and those needs associated with his role as a family person?

The correct answer is: (D) Give him writing materials so that he can write to his two sons.

In a bid to help this patient, the CNA can help him reach out to his two sons by providing him with writing materials. The scenario indicates the patient could have issues of belonging and probable doubts regarding whether or not he is loved. The medical staff, especially the CNA, should not neglect such needs. Although CNAs can assist such patients by ensuring they get access to writing material, they should not take it upon themselves to mail the letters. That responsibility should be left to the nurse, who will evaluate the letters and screen them first for appropriateness.

(41) It is the right of patients and their families to benefit from care _____.

The correct answer is: (C) That is culturally suitable for them.

It is important to consider the individuality of patients and their families when it comes to issues like culture. It is not appropriate to ignore the values and taboos in respective cultures when making decisions pertaining to health care. Moreover, individuals are within their rights to determine the lifestyle they want and what values to uphold. In short, in the course of providing health care, CNAs and other medical staff need to take into account and respect the personal values and beliefs of individual patients as they pertain to culture and religion.

(42) There are certain things medical staff needs to do at different stages of patient's treatment. In the case of a patient who is close to death, the CNA should _____.

The correct answer is: (A) Help the patient have peaceful final days.

When a patient is about to die, the main focus of the CNA is to ensure the most comfort possible, not only physiologically but also psychologically. It is incumbent upon the CNA to try and make the patient's last moments peaceful and dignified. As a CNA you need to help the patient come to terms with the reality of the situation, specifically that health is failing fast. The patient should also be allowed to exercise control over the remaining period of his or her life.

(43) Sometimes patients who have a terminal disease refuse to believe they are faced with imminent loss and can feign cheerfulness. This stage of the grieving process is referred to as _____.

The correct answer is: (C) Denial.

If a patient who has been informed he or she is facing a serious health problem that is deteriorating at a fast rate seems to still be very happy, that patient may be going through the denial stage, the first stage of grief, refusing to internalize the seriousness of the situation because it is difficult to deal with. Anger (not mentioned in the answer options) is the second stage of the grieving process. After trying to mask the pain of the reality in the first stage of denial, anger begins to set in as that mask wears off. Different people express their anger differently, some directing it to people closest to them. Sometimes patients direct their anger to their physicians for not being able to heal them. Bargaining is the third stage in the grieving process. During this period, the patient may begin to feel guilty about things in the past. Depression is the fourth grieving stage, whereby the patient goes through a period of depression after realizing there is nothing he or she is able to do to correct the sad state of affairs. During this stage patients feel bad about their helplessness and may discuss this freely with people close to them or those providing support. However, other patients in this stage of depression tend to withdraw from everyone.

Acceptance is the last grieving stage, whereby the patient has already come to terms with the reality of loss. Often patients at this grieving stage are not much interested in having people provide them with support and don't care much about their surroundings. If anything they often wish to be left alone to make their personal plans.

(44) In a bid to respect a patient's values including those of a cultural nature, you may wish to include foods commonly valued in the patient's community. If you want to show cultural sensitivity when caring for a Hispanic patient, you might incorporate _____ in the patient's meals.

The correct answer is: (B) Beans as well as tortillas

Beans and tortillas are food staples among many Hispanics. However, you should always check to ensure the patient does actually like those foods and not just provide them without asking.


(45) A CNA wants to interview a patient who is 93 years of age. Which of the following is the most suitable interviewing technique?

The correct answer is: (D) Speaking in a low-pitched voice.

It is important to keep in mind that this question does not indicate that the patient is hard of hearing. At the same time, it is worth remembering that for elderly people whose hearing is normal, exposure to loud sounds can be disturbing. At their age, they are often sensitive to loud noises or sounds. So you need to speak in a voice that is low in pitch as opposed to shouting. Since the 93-year-old patient has no other problem, there is no need for the CNA to use pictures to reinforce the message conveyed verbally. As for enunciation of words, it should be done as clearly with the patient as it is for anyone else. Poor enunciation of words can confuse any person, irrespective of their age. For example, if the CNA tells the patient she is going to come in with a 'pin' when what she means is a 'bin,' this may be worrying for the patient who might wonder which part of the body the CNA is going to prick and why. It would be as confusing to the elderly patient as it would be for someone whose friend orders her 'flies' instead of 'fries' in a restaurant. Good communication requires that you use proper intonation irrespective of the person you are addressing, and as for varying intonation, it helps to keep the listener alert when the speech being delivered is particularly lengthy.

(46) A 68-year-old woman patient has been diagnosed with colon cancer. The woman has daughters with the power of attorney, and they have demanded that their mother not be told of her diagnosis. After the daughters have left, the woman asks the CNA about her illness and diagnosis. Which of the following is the best answer for the CNA to give?

The correct answer is: (C) I promise to check out what is happening and get back to you. For now though, I have no information.

The CNA normally spends more time with patients than any other member of staff. As such it is important that he or she remain credible in the eyes of the patient. For this reason, it is inappropriate to lie to the patient. It is fine for the CNA to say he or she is not privy to the information as there is no shame in not having all information at all times, and it is believable especially when the CNA promises to make a point of finding out.

In reality, the CNA will be aware of the nature of the patient's illness and so giving the response suggested in options (B) and (D) would be wrong. It is bad to tell the patient she is in good shape when the truth is that the illness she has is serious and life-threatening. At the same time, the answer in option (A) is not a good one because patients are expected to communicate their concerns to the CNAs caring for them and not wait until the doctor pays them a visit.

It is also inappropriate for the CNA to declare he or she has no information pertaining to the patient's illness as suggested in option and still show no interest in finding out, as suggested in option (D), and so when you promise patients to find out things and follow through, consider that as buying yourself time to consult with your seniors. Communicate with your supervisor about what answer to give the patient. After that, return to the patient and fulfill your promise as that will ensure the patient continues to trust you, which is important with you being her caregiver. It is wrong to promise the patient something and then deliberately fail to fulfill it as that can break the trust necessary between the patient and the CNA.

(47)  A patient who has been in a long-term health care facility for a year tells the CNA, "I can't even talk with you considering how depressed I am. Just forget about me." Which of the following is the most appropriate response?

The correct answer is: (A) I'll stay right here in the room with you for a while.

Just because a patient tells you he or she doesn't want to speak with you is no reason for you to leave. You can't tell if the reason the patient has suicidal thoughts going through his or her mind and therefore wants to be alone in order to attempt suicide. Keeping that in mind, you need to remain close to the patient whether he or she speaks to you or not.

You can observe your patient in silence while studying the body language and general environment. When the patient speaks to you, make sure you actively listen for tone, nuance, etc. Be careful not to pressure the patient to talk to you. Instead, you should accept the silence until the patient wants to voluntarily speak to you. At the same time, let the patient know both in words and body language that you are ready to listen and to have a conversation whenever he or she is ready.

(48)  Suppose a patient you are taking care of says to you, "I feel worthless. I should not even be alive." Which of the following is the most appropriate response?

The correct answer is: (C) What is it that gives you that feeling of worthlessness?

Often people who are depressed have intense emotions that overwhelm them, and they react badly when they don't get a chance to vent and verbalize their emotions. It's beneficial to get the person talking about his or her feelings, and that is what you encourage when you pose a question like the one suggested in option (C). Once the patient begins to open up, you should keep encouraging him or her to tell you more with regards to his or her feelings. When depressed patients speak out, there is some relief they experience that is good for their mental and emotional health. This is not the time for the CNA to introduce new ideas to the patient. On the contrary, it is time to provide validation for the patient's intense feelings. It is important that the CNA listen keenly as the patient describes the feelings, and also provide encouragement. At the end of the day, the patient is bound to feel better because of the opportunity to have someone who both listens and is encouraging. Many times people think they are helping when they try to suggest solutions to the person's source of frustrations, and sometimes what they provide are common clichés. Such responses or suggested quick fixes serve to undermine the patient's feelings, and other times they end up making the patient feel even more worthless. As such, the CNA should refrain from offering solutions to the patient, and instead offer a listening ear and general encouragement.

(49) A hearing impaired patient is taken to the hospital and the unit where he is admitted is very busy. People with hearing impairments can suffer sensory overload. Which of the following interventions is appropriate to prevent this from happening?

The correct answer is: (D) Make a point of conversing with the patient from his bedside.

It is important that you converse with the hearing impaired patient from close proximity and direct any questions and suggestions to him personally. This helps to eliminate other disturbances and distractions as the patient has his full focus on you and your communication. This is also advantageous for the patient in that it reduces the chances of becoming overstimulated. As for overhead lights remaining on, this is a bad suggestion as it can cause a visual overload. It is also not good to allow family members to remain behind at will since if several people stay around it can add to the sensory overload the patient is already experiencing. Having the TV or the radio on will not help to alleviate or prevent the patient's sensory overload.

(50) Which of the following is accurate pertaining to patients' charts?

The correct answer is: (A) Patients' charts are the property of the hospital and nobody else should have access to them even on request other than the doctor who is in charge of the patient.

Patients' charts belong to the institution taking care of the patients, and how such charts are accessed is based on the institution's policies. So if a patient has been admitted to a hospital, his or her chart is the property of that hospital. Nevertheless, patients have the right to read their charts. However, they do not have the right to take the chart anywhere. They certainly are not allowed to take a chart out of the hospital. The only person with outright permission to access a patient's chart is the doctor treating that patient.

Patients' charts are not government property although they can be produced in court for evidence during a lawsuit, but proper procedures must be followed in such cases.

(51)  Jane, a CNA, has been charged with taking the vitals of a number of residents in a long-term facility. She carries out the task but fails to take the vitals of one of the residents. The nurse who oversees the CNA's work notices there is some information missing, and she asks the CNA about it. The CNA admits her error. The fact that Jane owned up exemplifies _____.

The correct answer is: (C) accountability.

Although forgetting to take the vitals of a resident when required to is a mistake, owning up to it when asked shows Jane is accountable. She has taken responsibility for the mistake, in which case it is easy to address the issue. The nurse now has a way of advising her on the best way to avoid forgetting any resident when taking vitals; probably a systematic way of doing it.

It is respectable behavior to own up to one's mistake, but there are several other ways of reflecting respectability. In any case, in this context respectability is not the best answer. As for flexibility, it is not the most suitable answer since it means the CNA's capacity to adapt to varying situations, yet in this case there was no new situation for the CNA to adapt to. Dependability is also not the best answer because in the case of the CNA it would have to be measured against the rules and standards set by the institution. In this case, what is being gauged is how Jane responds to her senior after making a mistake but not how competent she is.

(52)  Susan used to work as a CNA in a long-term facility, but she left two years ago to care for her newborn baby. For the last two years she has been a full-time mother, but now she has opted to resume work as a CNA to help pay increasing bills. What requirements will Susan have to fulfill in order to qualify to resume work as a CNA?

The correct answer is: (D) Retrain as a CNA and then go through the competency evaluation again.

The reason option (D) is the most suitable answer is that if you fail to work as a CNA for 24 consecutive months, it does not matter that you passed the evaluation test or have served for a long time as a CNA; you'll still need to retrain and get reevaluated for competency. There is no refresher course for CNAs that will exempt you from retraining and reevaluation once you have been away from active CNA duties for two consecutive years. That makes option (A) unsuitable. As for option (B), it is not recommended that you go straight for another competency evaluation without preparing anew. Option (D) is incorrect as the board would not accept recruitment of a CNA who has been away from work for an entire two years before retraining and retesting.

(53) It is a very busy Monday for the staff in your ward. The duty nurse hands you Terramycin ointment in its normal tube as she continues to prepare other medications for patients from the usual medication tray. She instructs you to apply that ointment to the eyes of a particular patient. What is the most appropriate response to her instruction?

The correct answer is: (C) Politely say that you are not authorized as a CNA to apply the ointment.

CNAs should always remember their roles and avoid carrying out tasks they are not authorized to do. If the nurse or doctor would like you to carry out a task that is not under your responsibilities, they should be beside you all along to do it under their instruction and supervision to ensure you do it correctly. Some of the duties CNAs are not expected to carry out include administering prescription medicine and applying medicated skin creams and ointments. They are also not expected to carry out orders directly from doctors or to perform procedures that the law prohibits. Whenever CNAs are not sure about a task, they should refer to the supervisor who is immediately above them in the relevant medical unit. CNAs should keep in mind that the motto of 'do no harm' applies to them also and not just to qualified nurses and doctors.


(54) A nurse who serves as a CNA's supervisor emphasizes the need for communication among members of the medical staff. The importance of this, according to the nurse, is to ensure care is given to individual patients in a manner that is coordinated and also effective. Communication by the CNA includes every one of the suggestions listed below apart from one. Which one is the exception?

The correct answer is: (C) Using terms that have several meanings.

Option (C) that suggests the CNA should make use of terms that have several meanings is inappropriate. In short, CNAs need to communicate using language that leaves no doubt at all in the minds of the people listening about the meaning intended.

(55)  A CNA receives a call while on duty only to realize the caller wants to speak to someone in a different medical unit. What is the best response?

The correct answer is: (C) The CNA should promise to redirect the call to the correct unit but also provide the person with the correct number in case the call is disconnected or the other unit's line is busy.

It is normal for CNAs to respond to calls coming into their units or in patients' rooms. It is important for CNAs to exercise good communication skills while responding to incoming calls, when calling other medical units or when redirecting calls to the appropriate numbers.

A CNA should not go looking for a nurse to attend to the incoming call because that will cause a delay. Delays in attending to calls in a medical facility should be avoided as they might be communicating something that requires emergency action. As a CNA you should find out the important particulars of the caller before trying to transfer the call, so that you can communicate that information to the person you are redirecting the call to. It is also important to keep in mind the need to transfer only those calls that you deem absolutely necessary; otherwise, refer the person calling back to the operator. Don't put the caller on an unnecessary hold if you are not going to be of help. Also, if you have gotten the gist of what the caller wants it is not a priority to ask about the number he or she tried to call.

(56)  You are working as a CNA in a long-term facility, and as you give one of the clients a bed bath a call comes in over the intercom. The unit secretary wants to alert the unit of an emergency phone call just coming in. The most suitable action for you to take is

_____.

The correct answer is: (C) Cover the client and put the call light close to him or her, then respond to the call. You have already been informed the call is an emergency, and so it is important that you attend to it immediately. You also have the option, though not provided in this question, of requesting that another CNA in your unit take the call. It is unacceptable for you to ignore the call. However, what you cannot do is simply dash out to take the call without considering the state in which you are leaving the client. You can't leave the door to the client's room ajar and the patient exposed, regardless of how important it is that you respond to the emergency call. The reason for covering the client first is to provide him or her with privacy and to prevent him or her from getting cold. In addition to covering the client, you should make a point of shutting the door behind you as you go out to answer the emergency call, or alternatively pull the curtains around the area you use while bathing the client.

(57)  In the facility where you are working as a CNA, you have received a new client. In order to facilitate proper care, you need some medical history pertaining to the client. This includes the nature of nursing support the client was receiving previously and what therapeutic management the client received before, if any.

The correct answer is: (D) Kardex.

Kardex is an information system used in the medical field, especially by the nursing staff, as a means to convey information that is important for patient care management. This system is concise and helps not only in recording data but also in organizing information so it is conveniently accessible to every member of staff involved in the care of individual patients. From the Kardex you are able to see information specific to the patient, which includes any nursing or therapeutic care that patient has received before. As for a flow sheet, its role is to enable nurses to make quick notes pertaining to an individual patient's nursing care, and it is concise enough to help one see how the patient has been receiving care and how his or her medical condition has changed over time. Progress notes detail how the patient is faring medically. You cannot go to the nursing discharge summary to seek information to help you care for an incoming patient, because this document is only compiled once the patient has been discharged from the facility.

(58)  It's time for the nursing round and as the team moves from one room to another they find a patient lying flat on the floor. Something must be entered in the patient's medical record. Which of the following is it most likely the CNA will record pertaining to the incident?

The correct answer is: (D) On entering the patient's room, the patient was discovered lying flat on the floor.

The reason option (D) is the correct answer is that it simply states the facts. As a CNA you should record only the facts available and refrain from adding your own opinion or speculations. As far as this question is concerned, there is no indication what might have caused the patient to fall. There is no mention of a probable cause. As such, you should stick to the facts without adding any details that you cannot substantiate; and in this case the fact is that the patient was found on the floor in a prone position.

(59) Patients' medical records are held at the facility in confidentiality. However, if staff members are not careful they can make mistakes that can compromise such confidentiality. Given that patients' records are computerized, what can put their confidentiality at risk?

The correct answer is: (A) Sharing personal passwords with other members of staff so they can access the computer when they can't remember their passwords

CNAs should avoid sharing the passwords they use to access the computers with other members of staff because once you have disclosed your password, someone else can use it to compromise patients' medical records. It is important to note that anything untoward happening because someone got access to records using your password becomes your responsibility. This means you will be the one who is assumed to have compromised the confidential records and the system access trail will provide evidence to that effect. It is necessary to maintain the confidentiality of patients' medical records at all times, including taking steps like the ones suggested in the other answer options. Logging out of all the computers you were logged in on is crucial. If you have access to more than one computer, you need to be logged out of all the computers apart from the one you are using at any particular moment. This will ensure nobody else can access patients' records using your access permissions without you knowing.

It is also recommended that you keep changing the passwords you use to access computers so that if you inadvertently expose your password to someone else they can no longer log into the system as you. As for denying someone unknown access to medical records, it's the right thing to do as you can't just take a person's word at face value. Just because someone approaches you and says they're a staff member doesn't mean they are. You can only allow members of staff whom you know to read the records you have.

(60) A registered nurse is taking you around for orientation in a facility where you are newly employed as a CNA. She informs you it is usual for patients from diverse cultures to be admitted to the facility, and some of them converse in languages other than English. What is the appropriate thing to do when faced with such patients?

The correct answer is: (D) Use an interpreter whenever you need to communicate with the patient.

It's best to have an interpreter with you whenever you are trying to communicate with a patient who does not understand English. Accessing an interpreter should not be a problem as the nurse who oversees your work can ensure there is one available whenever you make the request. The suggestion of speaking loudly and slowly does not help no matter how close you are to the patient, as the problem is not one of deafness but one of understanding. The patient can hear you normally like everyone else but cannot understand your words or your message because he or she doesn't speak your language. The idea of speaking to the patient in the presence of family members is discouraged not only because it does not guarantee you an accurate translation, if at all, but it also violates the patient's privacy.

# Test 3: Questions

(1) Giving a patient a bath is one of the most common tasks CNAs are expected to carry out, and so you will be expected to know the dos and don'ts of the job. Which of the following is an appropriate action to take?

(A) Make patients take a bath on their own irrespective of whether they do it properly or not

(B) Apply lotion on the patient's feet after the bath while ensuring the lotion gets into the spaces in between the patient's toes

(C) Ensure that all areas not being washed at any particular moment are well covered using a sheet or towel

(D) Clean the patient's perineal part by using a washcloth to wipe gently beginning at the back and moving towards the front


(2) Which of the following is a task a CNA cannot perform?

(A) Inserting a Foley catheter

(B) Helping a patient take a bath

(C) Informing the nurse when there is a patient with a soiled dressing

(D) Providing oral care to a patient who is unconscious


(3)   A year ago, a resident developed aphasia following a stroke on his left side. The term 'aphasia' is used in reference to _____.

(A)    The patient being confused

(B)    The patient not being able to hear

(C)    The patient not being able to speak

(D)    The patient not being able to void

(4)   Sometimes a patient with mobility problems might feel _____.

(A)   Laziness

(B)   Joy

(C)   Confusion

(D)   Sadness

(5)   There are regulations pertaining to the management of nursing facilities in the US, and one notable regulation is the Omnibus Budget and Reconciliation Act (OBRA). Which of the following indicates what OBRA requires nursing homes to accomplish for their clients?

(A)   Assist their clients to move to other nursing facilities if they so wish

(B)   Assist their clients to attain the highest possible level of mental and psychological functioning

(C)   Assist clients in their Activities of Daily Living (ADLs) and ensure they are not neglected

(D)   Assist clients in writing of wills as well as choosing powers of attorney

(6)   Which of the following patients will benefit most from the exercises described as 'range-of-motion'?

(A)   Patients suffering from depression

(B)   Patients who have hemiplegia

(C)   Patients who have a pulled leg muscle

(D)   Patients suffering hypertension

(7)   CNAs are expected to be reliable as they discharge their duties. Which of the following indicates a reliable CNA?

(A)   The CNA clocking in 20 minutes late

(B)   The CNA monitoring a client's vital signs

(C)   The CNA informing the duty nurse when a patient complains of being in pain

(D)   The CNA completing a task assigned to her by the nurse in good time


(8)   Patients and clients in hospitals and nursing facilities are protected under various professional regulations and legal stipulations. The Patients' Bill of Rights is one such example, and within it is the term 'grievance.' What does 'grievance' mean in the context of the Patients' Bill of Rights?

(A)   Patients should not call their doctors after they have gone home

(B)   Patients should be allowed access to information pertaining to their health at any time

(C)   Patients are allowed to file a complaint without being penalized or having any fear of repercussion

(D)   With regards to essential care, no monetary limit is set for a lifetime


(9)   Which of the diseases listed below needs no airborne safeguards or precautions?

(A)   MRSA

(B)   Chickenpox

(C)   Measles

(D)   Tuberculosis

(10)  As a CNA, there is a chance you will have to provide care to a patient who has Hepatitis C. You are expected to have basic knowledge about several diseases, and in the case of Hepatitis C you are aware there is a chance a Hepatitis C patient could have contracted the disease by _____.

(A)  Walking barefoot

(B)  Using IV drugs

(C)  Eating from dirty utensils

(D)  Sitting on dirty toilet seats


(11)  CNAs sometimes take care of clients who are depressed. One day a client who is seriously depressed tells the CNA he would like to commit suicide and already has a plan in mind, and that although he is unsure if he will be bold enough to do it, he still feels dying is better than continuing to live the kind of life he is living. What is the appropriate course of action for the CNA to take?

(A)  Report the situation to the doctor

(B)  Report the situation to the nurse in charge

(C)  Reassure the patient that the situation is not really that terrible and that he will feel better the following day

(D)  Ask the patient to elaborate on his feelings


(12)  There are instances where members of the medical staff are required to fill in details in a legal form. Which of the following may be used on those forms?

(A)  A red pen

(B)  A green pen

(C)  A blue or black pen

(D)  A purple pen

(13)  A CNA has been taking care of a patient known for her low blood pressure, and that patient is on prescription medication. At some point during the day the CNA takes the patient's blood pressure, and she is surprised the reading is 155/85. What is a probable reason for this significant change?

(A)   The patient has been lying in bed all day

(B)    The patient is under stress

(C)   According to the patient she has not skipped taking medication

(D)    The CNA tightened the cuff too much when taking the patient's most recent blood pressure


(14)  The difference between the left lateral position and the Sims position is _____.

(A)   When a patient is in the Sims position, the arm that is undermost is positioned in a lateral manner and is parallel to the body of the patient

(B)   When a patient is in the Sims position, a pillow is put between the knees so that they do not touch each other

(C)   When a patient is in the lateral position, the arm that is undermost is positioned in a lateral manner and is parallel to the body of the patient

(D)    When the patient is in the lateral position, the head is elevated at an angle of 15° using a pair of pillows


(15)  One of the tasks a CNA is charged with is helping patients move from a bed to a chair. Which of the following is *not* an important part of the sequence of movement?

(A)   Position a chair in the location that corresponds to the patient's strong side

(B)   Lower the bed as far as possible and lock its wheels

(C)   Help the patient into a robe and non-skid slippers

(D)    Encourage the patient so he or she can pivot with as little help as possible

(16) When it is time for a CNA to use a strait jacket on a client, it is crucial that
_____.

(A)   He or she applies a half-bow knot, securing every tie all around the frame of the bed

(B)   He or she ascertains that the client cannot hit other clients who are close by

(C)   He or she uses a square knot to fasten the vest ties together at the back of the client's chair

(D)   He or she ascertains that the client has room to expand his or her chest to allow for proper breathing

(17) Which of the following should a CNA report STAT?

(A)   If the patient's temperature has reached 98.9°F

(B)   If the patient's respiration rate is 32 per minute

(C)   If the patient's pulse rate is 72

(D)   If the patient's blood pressure is 102/75

(18) Which of the following describes empathy?

(A)   In a nursing facility, a CNA talks to a resident about his or her recent medical results that revealed he or she has cancer

(B)   A CNA offers to take a walk with a resident in a nursing facility or to watch a movie together

(C)   A CNA requests time off for lunch

(D)   A CNA discusses with the facility's dietician the need to change what is delivered on a particular resident's meal tray

(19) Instead of using the word 'convulsion,' one can also use the word _____.

(A) Hypertension

(B) Seizure

(C) Tremors

(D) Fever

(20) Which of the following is a good snack for a patient to consume at bedtime to get some extra Vitamin D?

(A) One apple

(B) Some pretzels

(C) A glass of warm milk

(D) One cookie

(21) Diabetes is a disease that affects one of the primary systems of a person's body. That system is _____.

(A) The cardiac system

(B) The respiratory system

(C) The endocrine system

(D)  The musculoskeletal system

(22) Among people who are 85 years and older, the most common cause of accidental death is _____.

(A)  Motor accidents

(B)  Poisoning

(C)  Drowning

(D)  Falls


(23) Which of the following is *not* known to interfere with bladder and bowel voiding?

(A)  Aging

(B)  Infection

(C)  Family-related stress

(D)   Medication


(24) There are three major things a CNA should take into account when preparing to give a resident in a nursing facility a bed bath. These things are a _____.

(A)  Resident's privacy, warmth and rest

(B)  Resident's warmth, cleanliness and safety

(C)  Resident's security, comfort and rest

(D)  Resident's security, privacy and safety

(25) Suppose a CNA who has been working for two hours since reporting to work feels indisposed and, on taking her temperature, realizes she has a 101°F fever. What course of action should she take?

(A)   Just continue to work since her shift is far from over, but wear a mask

(B)   Immediately stop working and go home

(C)   Inform the nurse in charge with a view of being allowed to go home

(D)   Continue working as normal but make a point of washing hands every quarter of an hour


(26) A CNA was close by when a resident in a nursing facility fell. She has been asked to write down what she witnessed, and it is expected her documentation will be acceptable for legal purposes. Which of the following has been correctly documented for legal purposes?

(A)   The reason the resident fell is because he ignored orders to remain in bed when I instructed him to do so

(B)   The resident slipped and then slid along the bedside to the floor, and ended up landing on his sacrum

(C)   The resident fell because the bed wheels were not locked as the nurse forgot to lock them again

(D)   Housekeeping had left bedsheets on the floor in the resident's room and he tripped over them and fell


(27) Which of the following medical disorders is irreversible?

(A)   Chickenpox

(B)   Hypertension

(C)   Asthma

(D)   Emphysema

(28) What does the abbreviation 'Rx' stand for?

(A)  A type of disease

(B)  Treatment

(C)  Acute ailment

(D)  A kind of wound

(29) If a CNA is taking care of diabetic patients, there are some symptoms that should be reported immediately when observed. One of these symptoms is _____.

(A)  A cough

(B)  Emesis

(C)  Bowel movement

(D)  Refusing to consume dessert

(30) Hand sanitizers are great for hygiene. However, some sanitizers should be selectively used. For example, a hand sanitizer that is alcohol based is inappropriate for use _____.

(A)   In a situation where the CNA has just come from a resident's room

(B)   In a situation where the CNA is just about to go into a resident's room

(C)   In a situation where the CNA is about to assist a resident to the bathroom and has gloves on

(D)   In a situation where the CNA's hands are visibly soiled

(31) CNAs are expected to know when urine color is and isn't normal. Normally a person's urine should look _____.

(A)   Pale yellow and clear

(B)   Dark yellow

(C)   Dark and have a foul smell

(D)   Dark yellow and clear


(32) A CNA wants to assist a resident in her unit to use the urinal. In order to accord the resident privacy, the CNA pulls the curtains to enclose the resident's bed within. It is all right if she remains on the outside of the enclosed area and tells the resident _____.

(A)   To inform her later in the day of the number of ml he produced

(B)   She will return later to empty the urinal

(C)   To call her in case he requires assistance

(D)   To call her once he is through so she can come and empty the urinal


(33) A resident at a long-term nursing facility is receiving bowel training. CNAs are expected to understand that people _____.

(A)   Receive bowel training in order to maintain their digestive tract strong and healthy

(B)   No longer receive bowel training under any circumstances

(C)   Receive bowel training when they have colostomies in order to help them develop a regular pattern

(D)    Receive bowel training as a technique to enable them to use the bathroom without the need to push

(34) Different illnesses have different symptoms, and just by observing certain signs a CNA can suspect the problem a patient is experiencing. Which of the options listed here below would make a CNA suspect the patient has a problem with swallowing?

(A)  Extremely slow chewing

(B)  Tendency to pocket food

(C)  Uneven chewing

(D)  Taking a quarter of an hour to eat a plate of food


(35) Sometimes a CNA might notice some bleeding close to the site of an IV as she takes care of a patient. What should the CNA do?

(A)  Report the observation immediately to the nurse in charge of the patient

(B)  Immediately clamp the patient's IV catheter and then inform the nurse about it

(C)  Remember to inform the nurse in charge next time she passes by

(D)  Report the observation immediately to the unit supervisor


(36) Although temperature is usually taken orally, for some patients it may be taken rectally. Often when rectal temperature is taken, it is because the patient is _____.

(A)  Anxious

(B)  Combative

(C)  Confused

(D)  Unconscious

(37) Typically blood pressure is taken from the patient's upper arm. Nevertheless, there are instances where blood pressure should not be taken from that part of the body if _____.

(A)   The patient has had heart failure

(B)   The patient complains that the process has been done five times that day already

(C)   The lymph nodes have been removed in the area surrounding the left arm's axilla

(D)   The patient has an IV catheter on either arm


(38) Communication is important whether it is among members of the medical staff, CNAs and their patients or between CNAs and patient family members. Although speaking is the most common form of communication, sometimes communication is accomplished non-verbally. Which of the following represents non-verbal communication?

(A)   Minimal facial expressions

(B)   Whispers

(C)   Use of hand gestures

(D)   Using words


(39) Which of the following exemplifies emotional liability?

(A)   A patient expresses happiness to the nurse and soon after shows signs of being upset

(B)   A patient who prefers a certain color is upset when she receives food on a different-colored plate

(C)   A patient is upset towards the end of the day and attributes that to exhaustion

(D)   A patient is upset after receiving news of having been diagnosed with cancer

(40) Which of the following most accurately describes the role of an ombudsman at a nursing facility?

(A)   Taking care of residents as though they were part of his or her own personal family

(B)   Investigating complaints raised by residents and then drawing the attention of the relevant authorities to those complaints.

(C)   Making residents as happy as possible

(D)   Assisting residents in setting up insurance claims


(41) At a long-term nursing home, one of the residents decides to enroll in one of the available afternoon activities. As a CNA, which of the activities listed below would you recommend for the 86-year-old resident?

(A)   Basketball

(B)   Gardening

(C)   Watching television

(D)   Tai chi with meditation


(42) A CNA is expected to be familiar with terminologies used often in patient care. Which of the following means the same thing as 'pulse deficit'?

(A)   Strong pulse

(B)   No pulse

(C)   The variation that exists between a person's diastolic and systolic blood pressure

(D)   The variation that exists between a person's radial and apical pulse

(43) A nurse is teaching a client in her unit about heart failure, and the more she teaches, the more confused the client appears. Which of the following is the best strategy to use with regards to teaching clients about heart failure?

(A) Provide clients with brochures with information on heart failure

(B) Provide clients with DVDs containing information on heart failure

(C) Encourage clients to engage in conversation with nurses on the topic of heart failure with a view to gaining a better understanding of the illness

(D) Instruct clients to repeat everything the nurses say to them regarding heart failure


(44) As a CNA you are taking care of a resident who has AIDS. You know that any resident with AIDS requires _____ precautions.

(A) Standard

(B) Contact

(C) Droplet

(D) Respiratory


(45) You are a CNA working in a long-term nursing facility and one day you deliver a lunch tray to a resident. You notice that before the resident answers any question you ask, he asks you to say it again. Knowing that just a couple of days before the resident had a fall, you decide there may be a need for you to take some action. What is the most appropriate step to take?

(A) Check the resident's head for bruises

(B) Report your observation about the resident's forgetfulness to the nurse

(C) Immediately take the resident's temperature to see if it is abnormally high

(D) Don't take any action now; the resident is only being forgetful

(46) A client has difficulty chewing ordinary food during dinner. For that reason, the best food for the CNA to recommend for the next meal order is _____.

(A) Pureed

(B) Soft

(C) A bit hard

(D) Liquid


(47) A patient in a nursing home has just informed the CNA that she expects a visitor outside of official visiting hours. The patient then asks the CNA if the visitor can be accommodated at the irregular time. The best course of action for the CNA is _____.

(A) To say, "Of course! That should not be a problem"

(B) To say, "I'm afraid we can't operate outside our policy"

(C) To discuss the issue with the nurse in charge

(D) To tell the patient to wait and see but do nothing in the meantime


(48) When administering an enema it is very important that the CNA _____.

(A) Review the entire procedure with the patient and explain what is expected to happen

(B) Assemble all the materials required in the procedure beforehand

(C) Open the window in the patient's room

(D) Reassure the patient that the procedure doesn't hurt a lot

(49) It's normal for CNAs to make a patient's bed. When it is time to make the bed, it is important that the CNA _____.

(A)   Straighten the bedsheets so as to reduce chances of wrinkles

(B)   Inspect the sheets for softness

(C)   Only use linen in the patient's room

(D)   Replace the pillow cover every four hours


(50) When a person is injured, rehabilitation care should start _____.

(A)   When the family takes the patient to a long-term nursing facility

(B)   As soon as possible

(C)   A few days after the patient has recovered from the injury

(D)   When the physician issues such instructions


(51) As a CNA, if you ever suspect a particular resident is being subjected to abuse by a person within the facility you should immediately report your suspicions to _____.

(A)   The facility CEO

(B)   The nurse who provides care to the patient

(C)   The nurse in charge of the unit

(D)    A co-worker who is also a CNA

(52) You are working in a long-term nursing facility as a CNA and one day you notice the resident you are about to give a bed bath has very cold fingers on his left arm which is in a cast. The action you should take is _____

(A)  Ask the client to tell you if there is pain in the fingers of his left hand

(B)  Provide the client with gloves to keep the hands warm

(C)  Immediately report the condition to the nurse

(D)  Immediately touch the fingers on the client's right hand

(53) Suppose one of the residents in your unit in a long-term nursing facility declares he is going to leave immediately and that nobody should dare stop him. What is the best course of action?

(A)  Tell the patient he can't leave

(B)  Advise the patient that the best thing to do is to follow the doctor's instructions

(C)  Ask the patient to be a little more patient and wait to see if the care at the facility seems more appealing as he gets better

(D)  Advise the resident to wait for the nurse so that he can sign some paperwork before leaving

(54) At the unit where you are working as a CNA, one of the patients is complaining that as he coughs he is discharging secretions that are thick and sticky, and you already know the patient has a respiratory disease. Therefore, you recommend _____.

(A)  That he walk outside to breathe some fresh air

(B)  That he try to produce a stronger cough.

(C)  That he cough as hard as he can at hourly intervals

(D)  That he drink a lot of fluids

(55) A CNA is taking care of a resident with a fever, and in the resident's words, he is feeling quite uncomfortable. The best thing for the CNA to do right away to help this resident is _____.

(A)   To advise him to go and sit outside for a while

(B)   To administer Tylenol 500 mg PO

(C)   To give him a good back rub

(D)   To provide the resident with a cool washcloth for his forehead


(56) You are working in a nursing facility as a CNA and have just overheard the nurse tell a patient he has been found to have a 'bulging tympanic membrane.' As far as you know, this is likely to mean _____.

(A)   The patient has a viral disease

(B)   The patient is soon going to be in more pain

(C)   The patient's ears require more frequent cleaning

(D)   The patient has an ear infection


(57) A patient who has been in the hospital for around a week is paralyzed from the waist downwards as a result of a motorcycle accident. Unfortunately, he is refusing to take any medications the nurse gives him. What is the most appropriate thing to tell this patient?

(A)   Why have you refused to take medication?

(B)   You appear to be upset

(C)   No worries. Tomorrow will be a better day

(D)   Remember, the medication is for your own good

(58) A 53-year-old man has just arrived at the ER having been rushed to the hospital by good Samaritans. This man, who is said to be homeless, has a core temperature of 90.2°F, and the doctor says he has hypothermia. Going by how low the man's body temperature is, you know the body organ under greatest stress is _____.

(A)  The heart

(B)  The lungs

(C)  The ears

(D)  The liver

(59) You are a CNA working in a long-term nursing facility and you have just reported to work for your shift. It has struck you that you are in a group with no nurse assigned. What is the best action for you to take?

(A)  Complain about the lack of a nurse loud enough for people to hear

(B)  Volunteer to issue medications to residents with the assistance of a fellow CNA

(C)  Draw the attention of the nurse in charge to the group's situation

(D)  Start to immediately identify the medications you are going to issue

(60) You are giving a bed bath to a patient when you notice he has some redness on the coccyx but the area is intact. The patient's condition is best described as _____.

(A)  Stage 1 ulceration

(B)  Stage 2 ulceration

(C)  Stage 3 ulceration

(D)  Stage 4 ulceration

# Test 3: Answers & Explanations

(1) Giving a patient a bath is one of the common tasks CNAs are expected to carry out, and so you will be expected to know the dos and don'ts of that task. Which of the following is an appropriate action to take?

The correct answer is: (C) Ensure that all areas not being washed at any particular moment are well covered using a sheet or towel

It is very important that you cover the areas of the body that you are not cleaning for the sake of warmth and privacy. This is why option (C) is the correct answer. The suggestion that you should make patients wash themselves irrespective of how they do it is erroneous. While it is healthy to have the patients participate in tasks related to their daily living such as taking a bath, it is inappropriate to let them do a bad job of bathing or feeding themselves and not lend assistance. As for applying lotion in between the patient's toes, it is not appropriate as it makes those areas susceptible to fungal infection. With regards to cleaning the patient's perineal part, it should always be done from front to back.

(2) Which of the following is a task a CNA cannot perform?

The correct answer is: (A) Inserting a Foley catheter

A Foley catheter is a urinary catheter and is supposed to be inserted using a sterile technique, which is a skill CNAs are not expected to have perfected. As such, option (A) is the appropriate answer. Helping a patient take a bath is normal for a CNA, and even those patients who attempt to bathe themselves can always be assisted. Informing the nurse when there is a patient with a soiled dressing is the right thing for the CNA to do as dressing a sterile wound is another task not under the responsibility of CNAs. CNAs can dress non-sterile dressing changes. It's also fine for a CNA to provide oral care to a patient who is unconscious.

(3)  A year ago, a resident developed aphasia following a stroke on his left side. The term 'aphasia' is used in reference to _____.

The correct answer is: (C) The patient not being able to speak.

Aphasia affects a person's language formation and comprehension, and it also interferes with reading and writing. The problem results from injury to a person's brain, and in elderly people like those assisted by CNAs in long-term facilities the cause is mostly a stroke. Nevertheless, there are some cases where patients have aphasia because they have brain tumors, have had trauma to the head or have a serious infection. While some patients with aphasia lose some aspects of language ability, others lose most of it and communicating with them becomes close to impossible. All the other options apart from option (C) are incorrect because aphasia has nothing to do with a patient's inability to hear or void and also has nothing to do with whether a person is confused.

(4)  Sometimes a patient with mobility problems might feel _____.

The correct answer is: (D) sadness.

The reason option (D) is correct is that patients who are immobile may feel sad and frustrated. These patients can't all be described as lazy. At the same time they don't feel confused as they understand exactly what is happening to them, and they probably don't feel joy either as a result of being confined to a chair or bed.

(5)  There are regulations pertaining to the running of nursing facilities in the US, and one notable regulation is the Omnibus Budget and Reconciliation Act (OBRA). Which of the following indicates what OBRA requires nursing homes to accomplish for their clients?

The correct answer is: (B) Assist their clients to attain the highest possible level of mental and psychological functioning. According to OBRA, nursing facilities should do their utmost to ensure their residents attain the utmost level of functioning, not only physically but also mentally and psychologically. OBRA also stipulates that nursing homes should enable their clients to make their own choices pertaining to their own lives. Whereas there may be CNAs helping clients as they prepare to transfer to different facilities, OBRA does not put any demands on nursing homes to help in such transfers. Helping clients in their ADLs is a role CNAs play as part of their duties and not as a stipulation by OBRA. In any case, helping clients in their ADLs contributes to their mental and psychological welfare. Assisting with writing wills and attaining power of attorney is not one of OBRA's stipulations.

(6)    Which of the following patients will benefit most from the exercises described as 'range-of-motion'?

The correct answer is: (B) Patients who have hemiplegia.

Hemiplegia is a medical condition where a person is paralyzed on one side. Although there are people who develop hemiplegia after suffering an injury to their brain, most patients become hemiplegic after a stroke where the brain is partially damaged by blood clots. Often the person with hemiplegia has one arm and leg damaged on the side, but sometimes the paralysis extends partially to the person's torso. In order to reduce the chances of more blood clots forming and damaging the brain further, patients with hemiplegia are supposed to take part in ROM exercises. These exercises are also great for maintaining proper functioning of joints.

(7)    CNAs are expected to be reliable as they discharge their duties. Which of the following indicates a reliable CNA?

The correct answer is: (D) The CNA completing a task assigned to her by the nurse in good time.

It is a sign of being reliable when a CNA completes any tasks assigned to her by the nurse within the expected time. When a person is reliable, it means they can consistently be trusted to do what is expected. Dealing with vulnerable people is very time sensitive, and staff at nursing facilities should be ready to attend to the clients in a timely manner. In short, nurses and doctors are happy when they know the CNAs at their facility are reliable.

Certainly when a CNA reports to work late she can't be said to be reliable, as she is expected to be available to assist residents from a given time. Failing to meet such timelines is a sign she can't be relied upon to be at hand when needed by residents, and that is a bad attribute. A CNA should monitor a client's vitals, but it doesn't necessarily indicate reliability. Option (C) about the CNA informing the nurse when the client complains of being in pain, while appropriate, again does not necessarily indicate reliability.

(8)   Patients and clients in hospitals and nursing facilities are protected under various professional regulations and legal stipulations. The Patients' Bill of Rights is one such example, and within it is the term 'grievance.' What does 'grievance' mean in the context of the Patients' Bill of Rights?

The correct answer is: (C) One patients' right is being allowed to file a complaint without being penalized or fear of repercussion.

It is the right of every patient to raise a complaint if they feel wronged or when they believe there is something wrong at the facility where they are receiving care. They should feel free to do so without being intimidated or threatened with penalties of any kind. The Patients' Bill of Rights actually encompasses several guarantees. The others include access to the patient's own health information, receiving fair treatment, having autonomy with regard to decisions of a medical nature affecting them and others. In this question, the word 'grievance' is the reason option (C) is the most suitable answer.

(9)   Which of the diseases listed below needs no airborne safeguards or precautions?

The correct answer is: (A) MRSA.

Methicillin-Resistant Staphylococcus Aureus (MRSA) is a disease that occurs when bacteria causes an infection. It is transmitted when a person's skin comes into contact with the skin of someone who has the disease. In short, MRSA is not an airborne disease, and so precautions like those taken to protect yourself from airborne diseases are not necessary if the threat is MRSA. MRSA is a hard disease to treat in comparison to diseases caused by other strains of the staphylococcus aureus bacterium. The reason for this difficulty is that the particular strain responsible for MRSA is resistant to many antibiotics. The incubation period for MRSA can range from one day to 10, depending on whether the point of bacterial entry on the skin is broken.

Although chicken pox can be spread when someone touches blisters, mucus or saliva from a person with the disease, the disease is also airborne and can be spread when an infected person coughs or sneezes near other people. As for measles, a highly contagious viral disease, its transmission is airborne and it usually spreads as people with the disease cough and sneeze, or simply breathe close to other people. Tuberculosis is an airborne disease and can be spread when an infected person coughs or sneezes near other people, or even when a person speaks or sings and discharges bacteria-laden droplets into the air.

(10)   As a CNA, there is a chance you will have to provide care to a patient who has Hepatitis C. You are expected to have basic knowledge about several diseases, and in the case of Hepatitis C you are aware there is a chance a Hepatitis C patient could have contracted the disease by _____.

The correct answer is: (B) Using IV drugs.

Hepatitis C, which is a viral disease, is serious and affects a person's liver. For some infected people, the infection may be acute but with proper treatment the virus clears from the system effectively. Hepatitis C is transmitted through bodily fluids, blood and drug IVs. When a person with Hepatitis C shares a used needle, the person using the contaminated needle may contract the disease. The disease is also sexually transmitted. The other three options—walking barefoot, eating with dirty utensils and sitting on dirty toilet seats—have nothing to do with Hepatitis C, because the person is not coming into contact with infected fluids.


(11)   CNAs sometimes take care of clients who are depressed. One day a client who is seriously depressed tells the CNA he would like to commit suicide and already has a plan in mind, and that although he is unsure if he will be bold enough to do it, he still feels dying is better than continuing to live the kind of life he is living. What is the appropriate course of action for the CNA to take?

The correct answer is: (B) Report the situation to the nurse in charge.

The patient in the example is suffering from serious depression. He has even become suicidal and the fact that he says he has a plan in mind shows the thoughts of suicide are so intense that they have put him at great risk. For that reason, the CNA should report the patient's condition and the particular incident to the nurse who is her immediate supervisor. CNA do not normally report to doctors and so option (A) is incorrect.
It is inappropriate to promise the patient he is going to be better, and worse still to allege the patient's situation is not very serious. Such a statement would only make the patient convinced that nobody can understand his situation and therefore there is no need to seek help. As for asking the patient to elaborate on his feelings, such a move might be helpful when the patient is only mildly depressed, but with a patient who has disclosed he has a suicide plan in mind, the option is not appropriate.

(12)   There are instances where members of the medical staff are required to fill in details on a legal form. Which of the following may be used on those forms?

The correct answer is: (C) A blue pen or a black one.

For a document to be considered a valid legal document, it must be written in either blue or black. However, given that most documents today are now typed, the distinction occurs in the handwritten signature. Although black is just as acceptable as blue in writing and signing legal documents, many people prefer to sign documents in blue because the rest of the document is usually printed in black. The contrast of the two colors, therefore, makes it easy for someone to see at a glance that the document has been duly signed. As for the other choices, red, green and purple ink are completely unacceptable.


(13)   A CNA has been taking care of a patient known for her low blood pressure, and that patient is on prescription medication. At some point in the day the CNA takes the patient's blood pressure, and she is surprised the reading is 155/85. What is a probable reason for this significant change?

The correct answer is: (D) The CNA tightened the cuff too much when taking the patient's most recent blood pressure

The blood pressure cuff contributes to results. If it's too tight, the blood pressure reading is exaggeratedly high, whereas if it's too loose the blood pressure reading is too low. As such, the blood pressure cuff should not be too large or too small for the person whose blood pressure is being taken, nor too loose or too tight. Optimally, your blood pressure should be 120/80, although it is not cause for alarm if it goes up a bit with explainable nonmedical reasons. People who are prone to high blood pressure include smokers, the obese, those leading sedentary lifestyles, the elderly, those who consume excessive salt, those who consume excessive alcohol, those under immense stress and others. Among those prone to low blood pressure are pregnant women, people who have lost excessive blood, those with serious infection, the malnourished and others.

(14)  The difference between the left lateral position and Sims position is _____.

The correct answer is: (A) When a patient is in the Sims position, the arm that is undermost is positioned in a lateral manner and is parallel to the body of the patient.

The Sims position is named after gynecologist J. Marion Sims, an American doctor who came to be referred to as the father of modern gynecology. Patients are mostly put in the Sims position when they are undergoing a rectal exam or enema. They lie on the left side and on their left hip with their lower extremity straight, and the right hip and knee are bent. Another name for the Sims position is 'lateral recumbent position.'
As for the lateral position, the patient normally lies on the left or even the right side. If it is the left side of the patient's body that is in contact with the bed, then that position is referred to as 'left lateral position,' while the position is referred to as 'right lateral' when it is the patient's right side that is in contact with the bed. Normally there is a pillow put in between the patient's legs to ensure comfort, including in the Sims position.


(15)  One of the tasks a CNA is charged with is helping patients move from a bed to a chair. Which of the following is *not* an important part of the sequence of movement?

The correct answer is: (D) Encourage the patient so he or she can pivot with as little help as possible.

Any time a patient wants to leave the bed and sit on a chair, even if that chair is just nearby, the CNA should offer assistance. Helping the patient to turn and move from one position to another is important to ensure an accident does not happen. Helping the patient wear a robe is important as it is a way of ensuring the patient does not feel cold, in addition to providing privacy. It is also important to have the patient wear non-skid slippers as they help protect from slipping and falling. As for placing the chair on the side where the patient is strongest, this makes it more convenient and easier for a CNA to help the patient, because the patient's effort to move is likely to bear fruit and that eases the burden on the CNA. It is also easier to get the patient off the bed when the bed is at its lowest level.

(16)   When it is time for a CNA to use a strait jacket on a client, it is crucial that
_____.

The correct answer is: (D) He or she ascertains that the client has room to expand his or her chest to allow for proper breathing.

The reason option (D) is the best answer is that in all circumstances breathing takes priority over other issues. As such, the CNA must ensure the patient's breathing is not compromised before addressing other matters pertaining to the jacket. Even the potential for the client to hit other clients in close proximity is secondary in comparison to allowing the client to breathe easily.


(17)   Which of the following should a CNA report STAT?

The correct answer is: (B) If the patient's respiration rate is 32 per minute.

The term 'STAT' is used in the medical field to alert staff that the situation is urgent and likely to be an emergency. The word is derived from the word 'statum' which in Latin means 'immediately.'

The reason option (B) is the correct answer is that a respiration rate of 32 per minute is high. Normally a healthy adult is expected to have a respiratory rate ranging from 12 up to 20 breaths per minute while stationary. As such, any rate that falls below 12 breaths per minute is abnormal, while any rate that goes above 25 breaths in a minute is considered too high. When a patient's respiration rate is either too low or too high, the CNA should report it to the nurse STAT.

As for body temperature, an adult is expected to be 98.6°F when normal, though as high as 99°F is acceptable. If body temperature drops to 97°F this is considered usual and no cause for alarm. However, if body temperature drops beyond 97°F or rises above 99°F, this is considered abnormal. A temperature of 100.4°F is considered a fever and should be attended to medically as soon as possible.

As for pulse rate, the range considered normal for an adult is from 60 to 100 beats per minute. For children ages six to 15, a normal pulse is 70 to 100 beats per minute, according to the American Heart Association. Blood pressure is considered normal at 120/80, but it is also acceptable if it rises to 130/85 or drops to 110/75. Blood pressure of 140/90 is referred to as high blood pressure Stage 1, and if it gets to Stage 2, 160/100, there is even more cause for concern. It gets worse at Stage 3 and Stage 4, where the rate has reached 180/110 and 210/120 respectively.

(18)  Which of the following describes empathy?

The correct answer is: (A) In a nursing facility, a CNA talks to a resident about his or her recent medical results that revealed he or she has cancer.

Empathy is the capacity a person has to appreciate the feelings someone else has, and to share those feelings. There is a difference between empathy and sympathy, with sympathy being shared between you and the other person and empathy being your own feelings towards the other person.
Discussing the sad outcome of the cancer test shows you have empathy for the resident. You are giving the patient room to release his or her feelings and showing you understand it's hard, because you understand if you were in his or her shoes you would like that kind of support.

(19)  Instead of using the word 'convulsion,' one can also use the word _____.

The correct answer is: (B) seizure.

A person who is epileptic can be said to have convulsions or seizures; they mean the same thing. It is also correct to say that not every seizure is a convulsion; seizures are varied. When a person convulses, their muscles contract in a manner that is uncontrollable, and this can go on for a number of seconds or minutes. Sometimes convulsions are confined to just a single part of the body. As for seizures, they release electrical bursts in a person's brain, and the part of the body where the signs occur depends on the area of the brain that has been affected by the seizure. Not all incidences of convulsions indicate someone is epileptic.

(20) Which of the following is a good snack for a patient to consume at bedtime to get some extra Vitamin D?

The correct answer is: (C) A glass of warm milk.

Milk is known for its richness in Vitamin D, and the same case generally applies to dairy products. As such, option (C) is the best answer. Although milk is rich in Vitamin D whatever its temperature, warm milk can help a patient relax at bedtime. Besides Vitamin D, milk also provides the body with Vitamin B2 as well as B12. It also has minerals that include calcium, iodine, phosphorus and potassium and is rich in protein. Pretzels are made out of wheat flour, and although they have some B vitamins like thiamin, niacin and riboflavin, they're not known for being high in Vitamin D. As for the apple, although it is rich in Vitamin C and has antioxidant properties, Vitamin D is not among its nutrients. However, it also has lots of fiber and water and would be a great snack for a patient at another time of the day. As for a cookie, it cannot be said to be rich in vitamins, let alone Vitamin D. Cookies are normally laden with carbohydrates and fat and are high in cholesterol. It is unlikely the doctor would recommend a cookie at bedtime for a patient.

(21) Diabetes is a disease that affects one of the primary systems of a person's body. That system is _____.

The correct answer is: (C) the endocrine system.

Diabetes affects a person's endocrine system and if not checked its negative effects will spread to other systems of the body. A person's endocrine system comprises several hormone-producing glands that regulate body metabolism and growth. Other hormones regulate a person's sexual function and reproduction as a whole, sleep, mood and other functions.

As for the cardiovascular system, it comprises the heart, lungs, and the circulatory system. The heart pumps the blood so that it can reach all organs of the body, the tissues and cells, and that blood serves to supply much needed oxygen as well as nutrients. The respiratory system is among a person's primary systems and regulates breathing. Breathing is not complete without oxygen being absorbed into the system from the inhaled air so that energy is produced and carbon dioxide eliminated, which is actually the by-product of that process. A person's musculoskeletal system comprises skeletal bones, muscles, ligaments, tendons, cartilage and joints. All these provide support to other organs of the body, as well as to connective tissues.

(22) Among people who are 85 years and older, the most common cause of accidental death is _____.

The correct answer is: (D) Falls.

Falls are the leading cause of death in people 85 years of age and above. People in this age group aren't prone to car accidents or drowning because it is rare for them to drive or go swimming. They are also rarely in the kitchen making their own food so they don't have much room to accidentally poison themselves. The onus is upon the people caring for the elderly to make their environment friendly and safe in order to prevent accidental falls. In a nursing facility, the elderly should be given non-slip footwear and their personal spaces should be uncluttered. Torn flooring, carpeting, etc. should be replaced immediately.

(23) Which of the following is *not* known to interfere with bladder and bowel voiding?

The correct answer is: (C) Family-related stress.

In the medical field, voiding or elimination is used in reference to the process of discharging waste matter from the body, and this includes excretion of feces and urine. Family-related stress is not known for interfering with elimination. However, elimination can easily be interfered with when an infection affects the digestive system or when a patient is on certain medications. Also, it is normal for the elimination process to change as a person ages. With regards to bowel elimination specifically, factors that can influence it include diet and intensity of exercise. For those who lead a sedentary lifestyle, bowel elimination is bound to be different from those who are physically active. Also, if fluid intake is insufficient a patient can develop constipation.

(24) There are three major things a CNA should take into account when preparing to give a resident in a nursing facility a bed bath. These things are a _____.

The correct answer is: (D) Resident's security, privacy and safety.

Security, privacy and safety are the three most important factors to take into account when preparing to give a resident a bed bath. Ensure every window and door in the room is closed. Cover the patient with something appropriate like a towel or a blanket as you assist him or her with undressing. The room should be heated to an appropriate room temperature as a room that is too hot or too cold will cause discomfort and also has the potential to make a patient ill. It is also important to ensure that the patient is well positioned so that there is no room for an accident.

(25) Suppose a CNA who has been working for two hours since reporting to work feels indisposed and, on taking her temperature, realizes she has a 101°F fever. What course of action should she take?

The correct answer is: (C) Inform the nurse in charge with a view to being allowed to go home.

Since a person's normal temperature ranges from 97°F to 99°F, the CNA's temperature of 101°F is abnormal. It is, in fact, approaching fever point. Since fever could be caused by infection among other things, it is only reasonable that the CNA should stop attending to the residents and instead take care of herself. However, it would be inappropriate to just abandon work and leave without reporting first to the supervisor, as the residents require someone else to attend to them. All these factors point to option (C) being the correct answer.

(26) A CNA was close by when a resident in a nursing facility fell. She has been asked to write down what she witnessed, and it is expected her documentation will be acceptable for legal purposes. Which of the following has been correctly documented for legal purposes?

The correct answer is: (B) The resident slipped and then slid along the bedside to the floor, and ended up landing on his sacrum.

The reason option (B) is the correct answer is that it clearly describes what happened to the resident, and it doesn't blame to anyone.
Option (A) is inappropriate as the CNA takes it upon herself to assign blame, which is unwarranted. In this statement, she assigns blame to the resident himself. Likewise, option (C) is inappropriate for the same reason, with the CNA blaming the nurse. In option (D), the CNA blames housekeeping for allegedly leaving sheets on the floor. In short, as a CNA, any time you are required to report an incident, you are supposed to write what you observed but not present your own deductions.

(27) Which of the following medical is irreversible?

The correct answer is: (D) emphysema.

Emphysema refers to one kind of Chronic Obstructive Pulmonary Disease, which usually causes damage to a person's alveoli—the air sacs found within the lungs. If you have emphysema, your lungs do not receive adequate quantities of oxygen, and you can experience problems catching your breath. There is also a likelihood of having a chronic cough and difficulties breathing whenever you exercise. The greatest cause of emphysema is smoking.

The other kind of COPD is chronic bronchitis, which causes chronic coughing. As for chicken pox, it doesn't last long and can largely be treated at home. When it comes to hypertension, people have been known to get rid of it by eating appropriately and exercising regularly, although some people continue to take some medication for the condition. As for asthma, some children outgrow it, while other people control the illness through bronchodilators and other medications.

(28) What does the abbreviation 'Rx' stand for?

The correct answer is: (B) treatment.

Whenever 'Rx' is used in medical records it stands for 'treatment' or 'prescription.' In the field of medicine, the abbreviation 'Rx' is used by physicians within their prescription heading. The term is said to have originated from the word 'recipere' or just 'recipe' in Latin, which means 'take thou.'

(29) If a CNA is taking care of diabetic patients, there are some symptoms that should be reported immediately when observed. One of these symptoms is

The correct answer is: (B) emesis.

Emesis means vomiting, and when it is observed in a person who is diabetic it could indicate a sugar imbalance. As such, immediate medical checking and treatment is required. That's why a CNA should report emesis in a resident to the nurse on duty. Still, it's important to realize that vomiting can be serious no matter the cause, because it can lead to dehydration. There is also the risk of aspiration when vomiting. In short, whatever the reason, any time a resident in a nursing facility is vomiting the CNA should report it to the nurse.

(30) Hand sanitizers are great for hygiene. However, some sanitizers should be selectively used. For example, a hand sanitizer that is alcohol-based is inappropriate for use _____.

The correct answer is: (D) In a situation where the CNA's hands are visibly soiled.

Hand sanitizers are gels, often with alcohol in them, meant to kill germs when used on your skin. A hand sanitizer comes in handy when water and soap are not readily available, but you should not use it as substitute for water and soap when those are available or when the dirt on your hands is visible. Instead, you should wash your hands with water and soap first and scrub them thoroughly. After that you can apply a little hand sanitizer for added protection against germs.

(31) CNAs are expected to know when urine color is normal and when it is not. Normally a person's urine should look _____.

The correct answer is: (A) Pale yellow and clear.

When urine looks clear and has a pale yellow color, it is an indication that the person is properly hydrated. Normal urine color ranges from pale yellow to deep amber. Urine is given its color by urochrome (also known as urobilin), which is the chemical responsible for the yellow pigment. How dark the color is depends on how concentrated or not that chemical is in the urine. However, in some cases the color of the urine is affected by certain medications, and also some kinds of foods that a person has consumed. For example, heavy consumption of beets, berries and fava beans can influence urine color. Whatever the case, it's important that the CNA note the variation of a resident's urine color from the normal so that an assessment can be done.

(32) A CNA wants to assist a resident in her unit to use the urinal. In order to accord the resident privacy, the CNA pulls the curtains to enclose the resident's bed within. It is all right if she remains on the outside of the enclosed area and tells the resident

_____.

The correct answer is: (D) To call her once he is through so she can come and empty the urinal. The reason option (D) is the correct answer is that it is the CNA's responsibility to empty the contents of the urinal after the resident has used it, and leaving to afford the patient privacy is appropriate. Option (A) is incorrect as it is not the responsibility of the resident to measure his own urine output. As for option (B), it is incorrect because the urinal should always be emptied immediately. Option (C) is not correct because the resident in this scenario is expected to be urinating and nothing else.

(33) A resident at a long-term nursing facility is receiving bowel training. CNAs are expected to understand that people _____.

The correct answer is: (C) receive bowel training when they have colostomies in order to help them develop a regular pattern.

Ostomy patients require bowel training because it helps them develop a regular pattern of bowel elimination. People using an ostomy bag particularly need bowel training because in many of the cases the surgeon will have removed a section of the patient's colon or rectum owing to illness or injury, and so the patient is not in a position to pass stool or release gas the normal way. Sometimes a colostomy irrigation is performed so that bowel movements can be better managed. Bowel training becomes necessary sometimes when constipation becomes chronic, or when a person loses control of bowel movements. During bowel training, patients are helped to program their bathroom visits so they're at the same time each day. This helps their bodies to develop a regular pattern of bowel movement.

(34) Different illnesses have different symptoms, and just by observing certain signs a CNA can suspect the problem a patient is experiencing. Which of the options listed below would make a CNA suspect the patient has a problem with swallowing?

The correct answer is: (B) Tendency to pocket food.

It is common for the elderly to have challenges when swallowing food, and while this is not unusual as people age, sometimes these challenges are caused by certain medical treatments such as surgery. Dental issues can also lead to problems swallowing. There are also cases where people face difficulties chewing and swallowing owing to health issues such as dementia, cerebral palsy, amyotrophic lateral sclerosis and multiple sclerosis.

There are several signs that serve as indicators to a CNA that a particular patient has challenges chewing and swallowing, and the CNA needs to be alert to the fact that such people are at high risk of aspiration or choking. One of the signs is pocketing food. Patients with swallowing problems are known to pocket food within their cheeks, other times beneath their tongue and sometimes even in the roof of their mouth. Other signs of swallowing difficulties include coughing as they eat, choking or excessive drooling. If patients eat their food unusually slowly, have teary eyes while eating or express pain when swallowing, these could be other signs of a problem.

(35) Sometimes a CNA might notice some bleeding close to the site of an IV as she takes care of a patient. What should the CNA do?

The correct answer is: (A) Report the observation immediately to the nurse in charge of the patient.

A hematoma develops when blood starts to leak from a blood vessel and enters the soft tissue in the surrounding area. Sometimes this happens because the IV angiocatheter has passed through two or more walls of blood vessels. Other times it happens when insufficient pressure is applied on the site of IV as the patient's catheter is removed. The CNA should report the incident to the nurse immediately so he or she can immediately act to correct the situation.

(36) Although temperature is usually taken orally, for some patients it may be taken rectally. Often when a rectal temperature is taken, it is because the patient is _____.

The correct answer is: (D) unconscious.

An unconscious patient cannot close his or her mouth around a thermometer. Furthermore, in order for the oral temperature reading to be accurate, it is important that the patient be in a position to breathe independently via the nose. Since an unconscious person is likely to have difficulties breathing through the nose, the rectal method is appropriate. Other common methods for taking temperature include putting the thermometer under the patient's armpit. Rectal temperatures are not suitable for the other categories of patients indicated in options (A), (B) and (C), because they would either resist aggressively or be scared of the process.

(37) Typically blood pressure is taken from the patient's upper arm. Nevertheless, there are instances where blood pressure should not be taken from that part of the body if _____.

The correct answer is: (D) The patient has an IV catheter on either arm.

Taking blood pressure the normal way—from the upper arm—is discouraged in this situation because doing so would impede the patient's blood flow intravenously.

(38) Communication is important whether it is among members of the medical staff, CNAs and their patients or between CNAs and family members. Although speaking is the most common form of communication, sometimes communication is accomplished non-verbally. Which of the following represents non-verbal communication?

The correct answer is: (C) Use of hand gestures.

Use of hand gestures is part of non-verbal communication. If a person also uses facial expressions and/or whispers, this is considered verbal communication.
It is important that a CNA be good at reading patients' non-verbal communication, because patients may be afraid to say some things verbally but could communicate these things non-verbally.

(39) Which of the following exemplifies emotional liability?

The correct answer is: (A) A patient expresses happiness to the nurse and soon after shows signs of being upset

Emotional liability refers to situations where people are not consistent with their emotions and switch from one extreme to another. In the example in this question, the patient is happy one instant and in the next the same patient is upset. Such a drastic change where nothing significant has happened in between is termed emotional liability.

(40) Which of the following most accurately describes the role of an ombudsman at a nursing facility?

The correct answer is: (B) Investigating complaints raised by residents and then drawing the attention of the relevant authorities to those complaints.

Just as in government, the office of the ombudsman assesses the validity of complaints raised and then draws the attention of relevant departments. The ombudsman does not work directly with the residents during investigations, and so there is not much room to care for the residents as if they're family. The same logic applies to option (C). It is also not the work of the ombudsman to help set up residents' policy claims or insurance claims.

(41) At a long-term nursing home, one of the residents decides to enroll in one of the available afternoon activities. As a CNA, which of the activities listed below would you recommend for the 86-year-old resident?

The correct answer is: (D) Tai chi with meditation.

At 86 years of age, the resident is at risk of falling and injuring himself. However, tai chi is a good exercise to help improve the elderly resident's balance, hence reducing his chances of falling. As for meditation, it has the capacity to increase the resident's happiness while lessening depression. Gardening is not advisable because it is a strenuous exercise for an elderly individual. As for watching television, it should not be recommended as it increases the chances of the resident developing stasis or sheer inactivity, which is not healthy.

(42) A CNA is expected to be familiar with terminologies used often in patient care. Which of the following choices provided below means the same as 'pulse deficit'?

The correct answer is: (D) The variation that exists between a person's radial and apical pulse.

The way to assess an apical pulse is by placing a stethoscope over the location of the heart. The radial pulse is assessed by placing a finger on the inner part of a patient's wrist and applying pressure with that finger as you count the patient's heartbeat. When you get the results of the two pulses and then subtract the smaller number from the higher one, the difference is the pulse deficit. All the other answer choices are outright wrong. The term 'pulse deficit' has nothing to do with how weak or strong a person's pulse is, and it has nothing to do with diastolic or systolic pressure variation.

(43) A nurse is teaching a client in her unit about heart failure, and the more she teaches, the more confused the client appears. Which of the following is the best strategy to use with regards to teaching clients about heart failure?

The correct answer is: (C) Encourage clients to engage in conversation with nurses on the topic of heart failure with a view to gaining a better understanding of the illness. If you want your client to understand a disease better, including how to heal faster, it's best to encourage client participation. This means they have an opportunity to say what they think the disease is about and the nurse has an opportunity to point out where the client has it right or wrong and why. When clients are active participants, their concentration is high as the nurse speaks, and they have an open mind and are ready to learn.

(44) As a CNA you are taking care of a resident who has AIDS. You already know that any resident with AIDS requires _____ precautions.

The correct answer is: (A) standard

The reason option (A) is the correct answer is that for AIDS patients you need to take standard precautions which include wearing gloves every time you handle bodily fluids, including blood.

Standard precautionary measures apply when you're taking care of any kind of patient, and they are, to a great extent, about common sense. You're expected to assess each case and situation and then decide what additional protection you need to take and what helpful gear you need to use for personal protection. When you take precautionary measures when caring for patients, not only do you protect yourself from infection but you also protect other patients whom you come into contact with.

Contact precautions are required when dealing with patients with infectious diseases like MRSA, RSV, open wounds, VRE, illness that involve diarrhea and other such ailments that can be spread through touch. In this kind of precaution, CNAs are expected to wear not only protective gloves but also gowns as they enter the client's room.

Droplet precautions are required when a patient is coughing and sneezing and has illnesses such as pneumonia, influenza, bacterial meningitis and whooping cough. Some recommended droplet protection measures include the use of surgical masks. Respiratory precautions are required when a patient has an infectious illness known to be transmitted in the process of respiration. Such diseases include TB, SARS and influenza.

(45) You are a CNA working in a long-term nursing facility, and one day you deliver a lunch tray to a resident. You notice that before the resident answers any question you ask, he is asking you to say it again. Knowing that just a couple of days before the resident had had a fall, you decide there may be a need for you to take some action. What is the most appropriate step to take?

The correct answer is: (B) Report your observation about the resident's forgetfulness to the nurse.

The reason option (B) is the correct answer is that often when someone begins forgetting things in an abnormal way and the person has had a fall, he or she has suffered a concussion. The fear is that the fall might have caused an injury to the person's brain, and that needs to be attended to immediately.

Option (A) is incorrect because a person can have a concussion even without sustaining any physical injury to the head. In fact, shaking someone violently can cause brain trauma. Option (C) is incorrect since having a high temperature or fever is not a sign that the person has a concussion, and likewise having a normal temperature does not preclude the person from having a concussion. Not taking any action as suggested in option (D) is wrong and might appear like negligence on the part of the CNA, especially since the abnormal forgetfulness is very obvious and the CNA is aware of the resident's recent fall.

(46) A client has difficulties chewing ordinary food during dinner. For that reason, the best food for the CNA to recommend for the next meal order is _____.

The correct answer is: (B) soft.

The reason option (B) is the correct answer is that soft food is easy to chew. Option (A) is not advisable at this moment because it does not require any chewing at all and it has not been established the client is unable to chew. Before ordering a pureed meal, the client should be advised to order soft food first. Ordering hard food, even if it is only a little hard, is not helpful to a client who is struggling with chewing. Liquid food is not required at this juncture when neither soft food nor pureed has been tried. Pureed food is food that has been cooked normally first and then afterwards ground, pressed and blended before being sieved into a creamy paste. Often purees are from vegetables and fruits or legumes.

(47)  A patient in a nursing home has just informed the CNA that she expects a visitor outside of official visiting hours. The patient then asks the CNA if the visitor can be accommodated at the irregular time. The best course of action for the CNA is _____.

The correct answer is: (C) To discuss the issue with the nurse in charge.

It's good to give the patient an answer in order to avoid anxiety on her part, but it's also important not to answer before consulting with the nurse in charge of the unit. The nurse in charge will make the decision after considering all factors including facility regulations and the patient's circumstances as explained by the CNA.

Option (A) is wrong because CNAs do not have the privilege of making decisions like these that involve doing things outside the standard stipulations. At the same time it's not the CNA's responsibility to decide if the patient's case can be treated differently, and so option (B) is also wrong. Option (D) is wrong as it is inappropriate for the CNA not to give the patient any answer at all.

(48)  When administering an enema it's very important that the CNA _____.

The correct answer is: (A) Review the entire procedure with the patient and explain what is expected to happen.

It's important to let the patient know what the procedure about to be carried out entails, and also what the patient should expect. It's also important that the CNA make the patient feel he or she will be treated kindly. That way the patient doesn't become anxious or panicky.

(49)  It's normal for CNAs to make a patient's bed. When it's time to make the bed, it's important that the CNA _____.

The correct answer is: (A) Straighten the bedsheets to reduce the chances of wrinkles forming.

Creased or wrinkled bedsheet can lead to bed sores because they exert friction on a patient's body. Bed sores are ulcers originating from pressure exerted on the skin. Bed sores vary in degree of seriousness, but often they are reddish and have some warm to the touch. As sores become more serious they develop blisters, and these can be painful and could break open. If not treated in good time, bed sores can cause infection.

(50) When a person is injured, rehabilitation care should start _____.

The correct answer is: (B) As soon as possible.

After someone has sustained an injury, the sooner rehabilitation can begin, the better for the patient's prognosis. Rehabilitation is often a slow process. Even so, there are many people who are totally immobilized by an injury yet after undergoing rehabilitation regain strength and in due course are able to walk once more, sometimes with the help of crutches and other times without any aid.

(51) As a CNA, if you ever suspect a particular resident is being subjected to abuse by a person within the facility you should immediately report your suspicions to _____.

The correct answer is: (C) The nurse in charge of the unit.

It is advisable to report such suspicions to the nurse in charge as she or he is in a position to handle such an issue effectively. Reporting to the CEO is not advisable as such an office is so high up the administration ladder that he or she will have to refer the case downwards for investigation and proper action to be taken. As for a fellow CNA, she would be as helpless as you are as far as taking action is concerned, and the only real help she could provide is reinforcing the idea of reporting to the nurse in charge.

(52) You are working in a long-term nursing facility as a CNA and one day you notice the resident you are about to give a bed bath has very cold fingers on his left arm which is in a cast. The action you should take is _____.

The correct answer is: (D) Immediately touch the fingers on the client's right hand.

The reason option (D) is the most suitable answer is that you want to assess whether the temperature of the client's left fingers is normal, and you can do this by comparing them to the temperature of the right fingers. If the two hands have vastly different temperatures it's an indication blood circulation has been reduced in the cold fingers, possibly by the cast. In this case you should proceed to notify the nurse so he or she can adjust the cast.

(53)  Suppose one of the residents in your unit in a long-term nursing facility declares he is going to leave immediately and says nobody should dare stop him. What is the best course of action?

The correct answer is: (D) Advise the resident to wait for the nurse so that he can sign some paperwork before leaving.

If a resident who has been receiving treatment at a nursing facility decides to leave before doctors decide it's the right time, he is required to sign an Against Medical Advice (AMA) form to show he is abandoning health care at the facility 'against medical advice.' If the resident does not sign that AMA form, the insurance could very likely refuse to pay the resident's cost of treatment. Sometimes the AMA form is also referred to as a Discharge Against Medical Advice (DAMA). According to statistics, patients who leave hospital AMA have a high chance of requiring readmission and are at a higher risk of death.


(54)  At the unit where you are working as a CNA, one of the patients is complaining that as he coughs he is discharging secretions that are thick and sticky, and you already know the patient is ailing from a respiratory disease. Therefore, you recommend

_____.

The correct answer is: (D) That he drink a lot of fluids.

The reason option (D) is the correct answer is that when the patient drinks a lot of fluids, the secretions in his respiratory system are lubricated, and so the patient is likely to find it easier to cough them out. At the same time, although it may not look like much, coughing and blowing the nose also causes fluid loss, and the body could do with some replacement. So when the patient drinks lots of fluids, not only are the phlegm and the mucus lubricated and made easier for ejection, but the body is also better hydrated.

(55)  A CNA is taking care of a resident with a fever, and in the resident's own words, he is feeling quite uncomfortable. The best thing for the CNA to do right away to help this resident is _____.

The correct answer is: (D) Provide the resident with a cool washcloth for his forehead.

Providing a cool washcloth is the best immediate action the CNA can take because, once placed on the resident's forehead, the washcloth is bound to make him feel a lot better. Of course, the resident also needs to be seen by the nurse because a high temperature is usually a sign of an underlying health issue, sometimes an infection; and if the resident is on medication the reason could be related to the known ailment.
Sometimes you can reduce discomfort from a fever with a bath, and that could even bring down the fever, but it's important to avoid cold water. The reason is that using cold water is likely to cause a person to shiver, and when that happens the body tries to compensate for that by generating more heat from within. That ends up exacerbating the fever rather than reducing it. Drinking lots of fluids is also recommended when someone has a fever.

As a CNA you cannot administer Tylenol 500 mg PO even if it might help because you are not authorized to prescribe medication for residents. Also, giving the resident a back rub or having him sit outside are not solutions to his or her discomfort. As such, options (A), (B) and (C) are incorrect.

(56)  You are working in a nursing facility as a CNA and have just overheard the nurse tell a patient he has been found to have a 'bulging tympanic membrane.' As far as you know, this is likely to mean _____.

The correct answer is: (D) The patient has an ear infection.

The term 'tympanic membrane' is used in reference to the eardrum, which is a thin tissue layer found within the ear and whose main function is to receive vibrations of sound coming from outside the ear and then to transmit them to the person's auditory ossicles. Ossicles are small bones within the middle ear, a part alternatively referred to as the tympanic cavity. When a patient's eardrum is bulging, ordinarily this indicates an infection. Nevertheless, the infection does not have to be viral; it could be bacterial. So there is good reason to consider option (A) incorrect. Also, there is no indication in the question as to why the nurse should predict more pain for the patient, and the reference 'bulging tympanic membrane' has nothing to do with pain. That makes option (B) incorrect. Option (C) is also incorrect as the term does not suggest the patient's ear was infected due to improper hygiene.

(57)  A patient who has been in the hospital for around a week is paralyzed from the waist downwards as a result of a motorcycle accident. Unfortunately, he is refusing to take any medications the nurse gives him. What is the most appropriate thing to tell this patient?

The correct answer is: (B) You appear to be upset.

The reason option (B) is the most suitable answer is that it prompts the patient to reflect on the reason for what he is doing, without making him feel judged. It also shows you are trying to understand the patient's position, and this can be therapeutic for him. The other options might make you sound insensitive or lacking in empathy.


(58)  A 53-year-old man has just arrived at the ER having been rushed to the hospital by good Samaritans. This man who is said to be homeless has a core temperature of 90.2°F, and the doctor says he has hypothermia. Going by how low the man's body temperature is, you know the body organ under greatest stress is _____.

The correct answer is: (A) the heart.

Hypothermia occurs when the body is losing heat at a faster rate than it is capable of producing, which leads to the person's body temperature dropping drastically to a dangerous level. Anytime body temperature drops to a level reaching 95°F as opposed to the normal 98.6°F, the heart goes into an arrhythmia, meaning it ceases to beat rhythmically.

The reason hypothermia is considered dangerous is that the body cannot function well at such a low temperature, especially the heart and the nervous system. In fact, if not treated quickly enough, hypothermia can be fatal. It can lead to heart failure and cause the respiratory system to cease functioning. Long-term immersion in cold water or exposure to low outdoor temperatures are common causes of hypothermia.
The other options are incorrect because those other body organs are only affected at a serious level after the heart has malfunctioned. So if a person with hypothermia gets medical care fast, the function of the other organs might not be adversely affected, though the lungs might be a little strained.

(59) You are a CNA working in a long-term nursing facility and you have just reported to work for your shift. It has struck you that you are in a group with no nurse assigned. What is the best action for you to take?

The correct answer is: (C) Draw the attention of the nurse in charge to the group's situation

You need to draw the attention of the nurse in charge to the fact that there is no nurse assigned to the group so that you can have a nurse assigned to attend to every resident under your care. After all, every resident requires a qualified nurse who can make medical decisions and issue medication. CNAs are not authorized to issue medications and so when there is no nurse around, the best course of action is to report it to someone senior; in this case the nurse in charge of the unit.

(60) As a CNA, you are giving a bed bath to a patient when you notice he has some redness on the coccyx but the area is intact. The patient's condition is best described as _____.

The correct answer is: (A) Stage 1 ulceration.

Option (A) is the correct answer because when the coccyx is red but the area is intact it is an indication there is ulceration in that area but it is still in Stage 1. Ulceration in this context simply refers to bed sore. Anytime the CNA notices a patient who has begun to develop bed sores, she should report this to the nurse.
Coccyx refers to the bottom of a person's spinal column, which is triangular in shape and bony.

# Test 4: Questions

(1)   The goal of rehabilitation and restorative care is _____.

(A)   Restoring a patient's rights

(B)   Restoring the main thing(s) the person cannot accomplish

(C)   Reinforcing the main thing(s) the person can already accomplish

(D)   Improving the whole person

(2)   You are helping a resident who is hemiplegic to dress. What is the correct way to assist such an individual to dress?

(A)   Start off by undressing the resident's upper extremity then follow up with the lower extremity

(B)   Start off by dressing first the resident's weak part or the extremity most affected

(C)   Start off by undressing the resident's weak part first or the extremity most affected

(D)    Finish by undressing the resident's stronger part or the extremity that is least affected

(3)   Mrs. Biswas is a 67-year-old resident at a nursing facility who has right homonymous hemianopia due to a stroke. In other words, her right visual field is adversely affected. As such, you need to be particular in where you place her meal tray. When positioning it before her, you should _____.

(A)   Ensure the food and utensils are within her left-side visual field

(B)   Ensure the food is all on the meal tray's right-hand side

(C)   Make a point of reminding her to check all over her tray to locate the food and utensils

(D)   Keep her company and periodically draw her attention to the meal, informing her it is positioned on the tray's right side, because otherwise you could be guilty of unilateral neglect.

(4)    What is one thing listed below that will not enhance the safety of your clients?

(A)    Checking to ensure all clients are wearing ID badges

(B)    Teaching clients a signal system

(C)    Assessing a client's capacity to ambulate before transferring him or her to a chair or bed

(D)    Always covering the client with three warm blankets at night irrespective of the weather


(5)    Which of the following is most likely to increase constipation?

(A)    Exercising excessively

(B)    Irregular bowel movements

(C)    Consuming contaminated food or water

(D)    Consuming a diet that is high in fiber


(6)    What measure is most appropriate to take with a resident who has fecal incontinence?

(A)    Assist the resident with elimination every two or three hours after meals and also use products meant for incontinence

(B)    Assist the resident with elimination every two or three hours after meals; give proper care to the resident's skin after elimination; use products meant for incontinence and also avoid giving the resident foods that form gas, such as beans, cucumbers and cabbage

(C)    Give the resident a bath before each meal; give proper care to the resident's skin after elimination; given the resident a full bath after each elimination and discourage the resident from finishing his or her meals

(D)    Avoid giving the resident foods that form gas, such as beans, cucumbers and cabbage

(7)   The doctor has issued orders that a resident who has an indwelling catheter be given bladder training. From the options listed below, choose the one that best describes the purpose of bladder training.

(A)   To ensure the resident voids in intervals of every three to four hours

(B)   To provide an opportunity for the resident to walk to the unit's bathrooms

(C)   To get rid of the catheter

(D)   To facilitate the resident's control of when he urinates

(8)   There is a new CNA in your unit called Rispa and the nurse has instructed her to take a patient's rectal temperature. Which of the following is a procedure you notice Rispa is following incorrectly?

(A)   Dipping a probe so that it's covered in lubricant for up to two inches

(B)   Telling the patient what is going to happen in the procedure and helping him lie on his right side

(C)   Asking the patient to take slow breaths and to relax while at the same time using the non-dominant hand to separate the patient's buttocks in order to expose the anus

(D)   Using the dominant hand to insert the thermometer probe into the patient's anus with utmost care while directing the probe towards the umbilicus

(9)   One of the patients just admitted to the hospital unit where Mary, a CNA, is working needs his blood pressure (BP) taken on an hourly basis as per the physician's orders. It is now 15 minutes to the next BP taking and Mary has noticed the cuff provided for use is not big enough for the patient's arm; meaning if used it will be too tight. If Mary uses this cuff, the patient's BP reading is bound to _____.

(A)   Be below the level of the patient's actual blood pressure

(B)   Be above the level of the patient's actual blood pressure

(C)   Be clearly inconsistent

(D)   Have a low systolic pressure and a high systolic pressure

(10)   Whenever you are providing oral care to a patient who is unconscious you need to be very careful to prevent fluid aspiration into the patient's lungs. Which of the following is most effective in preventing fluid aspiration?

(A)   Placing a towel beneath the patient's chin to prevent wetness

(B)   Washing hands and observing suitable control of infection

(C)   Putting the patient in a position where he is lying on his side while lowering the bed

(D)   Carefully cleaning the patient's mouth using oral swabs


(11)   You are a CNA working in a nursing facility and a diabetic patient is assigned to you for care. This afternoon you are preparing to demonstrate to the patient how best to take care of his feet. Which of the following is appropriate procedure for a diabetic patient to follow?

(A)   Avoid washing feet with mild soap

(B)   Weekly cutting of toenails and removal of cuticles

(C)   Soaking feet in hot water

(D)   Applying lotion on the feet to moisturize them and prevent dryness while avoiding the spaces between toes


(12)   Patients with Cheyne-Stokes respiration have been known to also suffer from apnea. How do you define apnea?

(A)   Respirations that are slow and shallow and at times irregular

(B)   The patient is unable to breathe when in the supine position and has to sit up in order to breathe

(C)   The patient stops breathing for upwards of 15 seconds

(D)   Taking abnormally long breaths

(13) The physician has ordered a colonoscopy for 52-year-old Amina Jones. Before ordering this procedure, the physician orders that Jones be given an enema for cleansing purposes. The position Jones should be in for the procedure is _____.

(A) Prone

(B) Sims left-lateral

(C) Supine

(D) Dorsal recumbent

(14) It is time to deliver Mrs. Don's meal tray to her room. Mrs. Don is a 68-year-old resident at a nursing facility and a stroke survivor who now lives with moderate dysphagia and a few neurological deficits. Which of the following is an incorrect statement to make about a patient with dysphagia?

(A) A CNA must always perform oral care on the patient before helping him or her eat

(B) The patient should be helped into the Fowler's or semi-Fowler's position because it helps minimize risks of aspiration during swallowing

(C) It's easier for the patient to swallow soft, pureed foods like custards

(D) There is no reason why the patient should be assisted when eating.

(15) A doctor attending a patient in a facility where you are working as a CNA asks for a pair of sterile scissors. There is one pair of scissors on a locker nearby that is still in its factory wrapping, but it is clear it has been opened and then taped closed again. What action should you take?

(A) Give the pair of scissors on the locker to the doctor

(B) Ask another CNA if the scissors on the locker are sterile

(C) Refer to the facility's manual pertaining to supplies that have already been opened

(D) Get a new pair of sterile scissors for the doctor to use

(16) Sometimes a physician may recommend a back massage for a patient. When you are giving a back massage, what is the best position for a patient to be in?

(A) The supine position

(B) Side-lying position

(C) The prone position

(D) Fowler's position

(17) When you are giving a bed bath to a client, the recommended sequence is _____.

(A) Face first, then arms followed by chest and then legs, back and buttocks

(B) Face first, then arms followed by legs and then chest, back and buttocks

(C) Face first, then chest followed by arms and then back, buttocks and legs

(D) Face first, then chest followed by arms and then legs, back and buttocks.

(18) CNAs are sometimes called upon to do some heavy lifting, and it is important that they protect themselves as they perform their duties. When trying to move a patient or a heavy object from one location to another, the CNA should keep the workload as close as possible to the center of gravity in order to prevent fatigue and muscle strain.

Which of the following demonstrates the best way for a CNA to carry someone or something heavy from one point to another?

(A) Position yourself as far as possible from the work location

(B) Ensure the person or object being carried is as close as possible to your body

(C) Ensure the patient's bed has been lowered as far down as possible and the rails on the side are up

(D) Ensure your neck and arms are hyperextended whenever that is possible as you relocate the person or object

(19)  Mrs. Rodriguez has a nasogastric tube. The normal position for Mrs. Rodriguez to be in when being fed, unless it is contraindicated, is _____.

(A)   Right lateral

(B)   Supine and also flat

(C)   Flat and with the head towards one of the sides

(D)   High Fowler's

(20) A resident in the unit you are working in has an infection that is bacterial and very virulent. Which of the following is the best precautionary measure to avoid the possible spread of the bacterial infection?

(A)   Droplet precautions

(B)   Protective precautions

(C)   Contact precautions

(D)   Airborne precautions

(21)  Janice is an elderly patient who has just been admitted to the nursing facility and brought to the unit where you are working, and she is a first-timer at the facility. Which of the following procedures will help ensure Janice's safety?

(A)   Maintain the bed's side rails always up

(B)   Ensure no furniture is in the way

(C)   Keep all pieces of equipment out of sight

(D)   Keep the light on at all times

(22) Mr. Castrol, aged 56, has chronic bronchitis. Which of the following will not enhance his respiratory function?

(A)   Reducing smoking of cigarettes

(B)   Exercises that involve breathing deeply and coughing

(C)   Sufficient intake of fluids

(D)   Frequent changing of the patient's position if the patient is bedridden

(23) Georgina is giving a patient a bed path when she notices the Foley catheter is no longer taped on the anterior part of the patient's thigh. Georgina decides to correct that anomaly by obtaining some medical tape and securing the Foley catheter back in place. The rationale behind a urethral catheter's lateral anchoring, otherwise termed upward anchoring, when it applies to a male patient, is _____.

(A)   It accords the patient privacy

(B)   It promotes the comfort of the patient

(C)   It helps properly secure the catheter

(D)   It helps ensure there is no pressure within the patient's penescrotal region

(24) Which of the following best describes the purpose of an enema?

(A)   To relieve the patient of gaseous distension

(B)   To provide lubrication for the patient's colon and rectum

(C)   To facilitate oil absorption into the patient's feces so that they become softer and easier for the patient to pass

(D)   To facilitate stimulation of peristalsis

(25) Irene is a CNA who has been working at a long-term nursing home for two years. At the beginning of her third year at the facility, a 70-year-old resident is assigned to her. As a CNA, Irene is expected to give the patient bed baths. Every time Irene gives the patient a bed bath, the first action she should take is _____.

(A)   To adjust the patient's bed so that it's not raised but flat

(B)   To begin undressing the patient from under the top sheet so as to ensure privacy

(C)    To close every door and window in the patient's room

(D)   To let the patient know she is about to receive a bed bath and explain the reason

(26) Patients on a clear liquid diet should not consume _____.

(A)   Popsicles

(B)   Broth

(C)   Ice cream

(D)   Gelatin

(27) Michelle is a 26-year-old office clerk who has been put under observation to determine whether she has an eating disorder. Michelle must be weighed on a daily basis. In order to ensure the daily weighing is accurate, a CNA should not _____.

(A)   Make use of the very same scale every time Michelle's weight is taken

(B)   Take Michelle's weight at varying times every day.

(C)   Ensure Michelle wears the same clothes whenever she is weighed

(D)   Make sure the scale is balanced at point zero.

(28) Which of the following should a CNA not do when taking a radial pulse?

(A)   Assess the patient's pulse rate and rhythm, as well as bilateral equality and volume

(B)   Use the thumb to palpate the artery

(C)   Ensure the palms of the patient point downwards

(D)    Palpate the patient's inner wrist using two or three fingertips

(29) In some unfortunate instances, patients develop pressure ulcers. Signs that mark the initial stage of these ulcers include _____.

(A)   Skin that is still intact but erythematic and non-blanchable

(B)   Skin that has partially lost its thickness and the epidermis, dermis or both are adversely affected

(C)   Skin that has completely lost thickness, damaging the subcutaneous tissue or causing necrosis

(D)   Skin that has completely lost thickness, tissue that has developed necrosis or damage caused to the muscles

(30) The symptoms of hyperglycemia include _____.

(A)   Becoming irritable, rapid pulse and excessive perspiration

(B)   Gaining weight, rapid pulse and feeling of tiredness

(C)   Feeling thirsty, losing weight and urinating frequently

(D)   Losing weight, developing diarrhea and abdominal pains

(31) Osteoarthritis can confine a patient to bed for long periods. As CNAs care for patients who remain on bed rest for prolonged durations, they should _____.

(A)   Ensure patients lie still during massage

(B)   Keep providing passive ROM while decreasing stimulation

(C)   Keep turning the patient every two hours while encouraging the patient to cough and take deep breaths

(D)   Keep encouraging the patient to cough and take deep breaths while limiting fluid intake

(32) Juma, a patient who was brought to the hospital three days ago, has just undergone surgery to repair his hip. It is therefore important to position Juma's legs and hips appropriately. The most suitable position for Juma is _____.

(A)   Adduction

(B)   Supination

(C)   Abduction

(D)   Prone

(33) Mrs. Simpson's left arm is paralyzed and she has been in the hospital for two and a half months due to problems feeding herself. Not surprisingly, she has been relying on the CNA to help her eat. Which of the following is an incorrect statement about assisting patients with eating?

(A)   Let the patient tell you the order she wants to eat her food in

(B)   Let the patient inform you if she would like to pray before she begins to eat

(C)   Engage the patient in pleasant conversation

(D)   Use a fork when feeding the patient

(34) Mr. Wong is a 64-year-old man who only recently emigrated from Singapore. Today he appears extraordinarily agitated. As the CNA assigned to Mr. Wong, which of the following is a good activity for you to suggest Mr. Wong partake in?

(A) Bingo

(B) Table tennis or any other competitive sport

(C) Taking a daily walk

(D) Personal hobbies


(35) The problem of stereotyping when caring for patients is that it could end up _____.

(A) Enhancing cooperation with patients and their family members

(B) Causing more frustration for the CNA than for the patient

(C) Causing less frustration for the CNA than for the patient

(D) Causing an erroneous medical diagnosis


(36) When feeding patients in a long-term nursing facility, it is always good to be sensitive to cultural preferences. Therefore when a resident of Indian descent is under your care, you might expect his diet to incorporate _____.

(A) French fries and beef

(B) Roti and pork

(C) Rice, roti and curry

(D) Tortillas and beans

(37) Suppose you enter a patient's room and he tells you there are bugs all over his bed and he wants you to get rid of them, but you see no bugs. What is the best response?

(A)   Please stay calm. You'll stop feeling the crawling sensation if you relax

(B)   I realize you're afraid and I'll keep you company although there are actually no bugs that I can see anywhere in your bed

(C)   Stop worrying. I'll get rid of all the bugs bothering you

(D)   There aren't any bugs. Your mind is tricking you.


(38) John, a patient who is confused, is under the care of Jean, a CNA who has five years of experience. Every night at 8:30 p.m., Jean takes John to the bathroom before assisting him in getting settled in bed. The routine established by Jean for John exemplifies _____.

(A)   Providing orientation cues

(B)   Establishing a consistent routine

(C)   Encouraging patient participation

(D)   Bladder and bowel training


(39) In the report made at the end of the shift, the nurse informs the CNA that Mrs. Bradshaw, who is Jewish, has requested a meal that is a strictly kosher diet, and the information has already been relayed to the dietary section of the nursing facility. Which of the following meals is most appropriate for Mrs. Bradshaw?

(A)   Crab salad on croissant, potato salad, vegetable dip and milk

(B)   Rice, vegetables and roast pork, bowl of mixed fruits and milk

(C)   Shrimp, vegetables, Fettuccini Alfredo, salad, bowl of mixed fruits and iced tea

(D)   Sweet and sour chicken, rice, vegetables, bowl of mixed fruits and juice

(40) As a new CNA in a long-term nursing facility, your supervisor is taking you around for orientation. One of the residents approaches you and addresses you saying he does not belong at the facility and pleads with you to get him out. Which of the following is the best response?

(A) Since I'm new and just being given an orientation, I'll come back and talk to you later

(B) I am in no position to help you

(C) I think such a complaint is best directed to the nurse in charge of the unit

(D) What do you want to do once you get out of this facility?


(41) Which of the following is a component in the communications process?

(A) Speaker and listener, reply

(B) Verbal, non-verbal and written

(C) Message and sender, feedback, receiver and channel

(D) Voice tone, facial expressions and gestures


(42) During his orientation at a new nursing facility, the nurse who is to be CNA Jason's supervisor emphasizes the need for CNAs and all staff comprising the health team to be well coordinated and communicate with one another in order to provide the best possible care to residents. Which of the following will not help enhance communication?

(A) Being brief and concise in communication

(B) Providing facts and being specific

(C) Presenting information in a logical, sequential manner

(D) Making use of terms that have a range of meanings

(43) Communication is considered ongoing, dynamic and is a multi-dimensional process. Which of communication's components is referred to as 'decoder'?

(A)  The referent

(B)  The sender

(C)  Feedback

(D)  The receiver



(44) CNAs are not licensed nurses, and although their work is very important in the health care sector there are some tasks they are not permitted to undertake. Which of the following is not a task you should refuse to carry out?

(A)  A task you have always disliked

(B)  A task you find yourself doing in the absence of your supervisor

(C)  A task not included in your job description

(D)   A task not within the legal scope of your duties as a CNA



(45)  Which of the following is correct about an advance directive?

(A)  An advance directive means the same thing as a Do Not Resuscitate

(B)   The doctor has already assessed the wishes as stated in the document with the intention of determining what the patient wants or does not want

(C)   This is a directive that can only apply to a patient who is able to understand and make his or her own choices

(D)   The patient's relatives are to be accorded legal rights so they can make decisions pertaining to his or her care

(46) Which of the following is correct about conferences held in a nursing facility?

(A) Residents in the nursing facility cannot attend

(B) Residents in the nursing facility can only attend on invitation by the physician

(C) Members of residents' families cannot attend

(D) Residents have room to refuse any of the suggestions the health care team gives


(47) Sometimes CNAs need to ask residents questions in a direct manner because there is some specific information they require. Which of the following exemplifies a direct question?

(A) You said you are not able to work

(B) What are you planning regarding going home?

(C) Are you feeling better this time?

(D) What do you plan on doing once you get home?


(48) Communication is very important in helping to provide care to patients, but sometimes there are hindrances or barriers to communication. Which of the following best exemplifies a barrier in communication?

(A) Exercising total silence

(B) Using universally accepted medical abbreviations

(C) Using an interpreter to speak on behalf of a resident

(D) Cultural variations between the nursing staff and the residents

(49) Agnes is a CNA at a nursing facility, and she has overheard a colleague speak of the nurse in charge of their floor being in an illicit relationship with one of the physicians. Agnes has decided to give this information to her supervising nurse. Which of the following is the best description of the situation?

(A)   Agnes has opted to participate in gossip and this is unprofessional behavior

(B)   Agnes has been eavesdropping and now wants to seek clarification of the matter from her supervisor

(C)   Agnes wants to have her supervisor intervene because the situation is scandalous, and the name of their employer must be protected

(D)   Agnes is just protecting a coworker against gossip


(50) Sometimes there may be a need to do a background check on a newly recruited CNA. The best authority to provide information of this nature is _____.

(A)   The CNA's most recent employer

(B)   The 1987 OBRA

(C)   The Nursing Assistant Registry

(D)   The NCSBN


(51) CNAs and other health care givers are expected to show empathy for their clients as they take care of them. Which of the following demonstrates empathy on the part of a CNA?

(A)   Putting the needs of other people before your own

(B)   Putting yourself in other people's shoes

(C)   Doing something extra for another person

(D)   Sharing your emotions with the residents you are taking care of

(52) The most suitable time to make use of a soft Toothette is when _____.

(A)   A client is experiencing seizures

(B)   An unconscious client requires oral care

(C)   A client has complained he or she is having a toothache

(D)   A client is wearing dentures


(53)   There is a resident in your unit who had a stroke a few weeks ago but is now recovering. His entire left side is very weak, and now you have been requested to assist the resident to put on a warm sweater. You should provide assistance to the resident from _____.

(A)   The right-hand side of the resident

(B)   The left-hand side of the resident

(C)   Behind where the resident is positioned

(D)   The front of where the resident is positioned


(54)   You are the CNA in charge of a resident who has Alzheimer's, and this particular day there have been a lot of visitors in his room who have stayed for several hours. Since it is now time for the resident to bathe, the most suitable action for you to take is

_____.

(A)   Request the visitors leave the room until the resident has completed his bath

(B)   Postpone the resident's bath till tomorrow morning

(C)   Request the nurse in charge talk with the resident's visitors

(D)   Ask the resident when the best time is for you to return

(55) There is a resident at the nursing facility who has been put on the DASH diet. The resident is eating less now and appears not to like her food. As the CNA caring for this patient, what is the best step for you to take?

(A)   Ask the facility nutritionist to intervene

(B)   Have a discussion with members of the resident's family to see if they can bring the resident some favorite foods from home

(C)   Talk to the resident and try to get her to eat more

(D)   See if the doctor has prescribed any dietary supplements and if so, make sure the resident takes them

(56) Jason is required to report for physical therapy every day after breakfast, but it has become a habit for him to get there late because he feeds himself and eats his breakfast slowly. What is the correct action to take in this situation?

(A)   Have Jason go to physical therapy before eating breakfast

(B)   Starting feeding Jason yourself

(C)   Motivate Jason to eat faster by removing the breakfast tray from him as the scheduled physical therapy hour approaches

(D)   Ensure Jason is served breakfast earlier in the day

(57) Which of the following is not a typical eating challenge that residents face?

(A)   Inability to manipulate eating utensils

(B)   Decreased capacity to recognize hunger or thirst

(C)   Problems when chewing or swallowing

(D)   Forgetting when mealtime is

(58) Bathing residents who are weak or bedridden is one of the tasks performed by CNAs. Nevertheless, there is one important aspect associated with a resident's bathing needs that caregivers often overlook or forget, and that is_____.

(A)   The need to make sure the bathwater is a safe, comfortable temperature.

(B)   The frequency with which people bathe varies from culture to culture

(C)   The importance of following recommended body mechanics so as to prevent injury to the resident during the process of bathing

(D)   The need to rinse the resident thoroughly before drying him or her properly


(59) Although there are some standard procedures followed when providing health care to residents, there are procedures that CNAs are expected to follow because of stipulations in a particular facility. From the procedures below, identify the one a CNA would follow because of rules at the nursing facility.

(A)   Toenail-cutting policy

(B)   When providing nail care to a resident, note any nail beds that are either pale or blue and report observations to the licensed nurse

(C)   Provide nail care to a resident when he or she is seated in a chair

(D)   Soak toenails for around 10 minutes before they are trimmed


(60) Many residents receiving care in long-term nursing facilities have dentures. Which of the following is a false statement about denture care?

(A)   When dentures are moist, they are quite slippery

(B)   It is very easy for dentures to break, yet replacing them is expensive

(C)   Dentures are supposed to be immersed in cool water for storage purposes

(D)   Taking care of dentures is the responsibility of the residents themselves, and for that reason there is no chance of charging the nursing facility with negligence if a resident's dentures are ever damaged.

# Test 4: Answers & Explanations

*Covering general topics*

(1)The goal of rehabilitation and restorative care is _____.

The correct answer is: (D) Improving the whole person.

The purpose of taking someone through rehabilitation and providing restorative care is to try and make the person whole again, so that they are able to go through life as normally as possible in all respects. The reason people require rehabilitation is that they presently cannot operate as they used to before their illness or injury. People who have had serious injuries or illnesses not only need to be able to function well physically, but they also need to regain their independence economically. They also need to be psychologically fit and able to fit in socially. That is what the process of rehabilitation is for—to try and enable the person to live and function as normally as is possible.

(2)    You are helping a resident who is hemiplegic dress. What is the correct way to assist such an individual to dress?

The correct answer is: (B) Start off by dressing first the resident's weak part or the extremity most affected

Option (B) is the correct answer because whenever you are assisting a resident who is hemiplegic to dress you should ensure the area that is weak is undressed last.
 A person is described as being hemiplegic if they suffer from hemiplegia, which at times is referred to as hemiparesis. This condition affects one of the two sides of a person's body, hence the use of the prefix 'hemi' that is derived from the Greek for 'two.' When someone is hemiplegic, one arm, one leg, one side of the face and all other parts of the same side are non-functional after a brain injury. When you are done removing the old clothes and must help a resident put on a clean set of clothes you should start off dressing the weak part or the extremity most adversely affected. All the other answer options have it all mixed up and that is the reason they are wrong.

(3)   Mrs. Biswas is a 67-year-old resident at a nursing facility who has right homonymous hemianopia due to a stroke. In other words, her right visual field is adversely affected. As such, you need to be particular in where you place her meal tray. When positioning it before her, you should _____.

The correct answer is: (D) Keep her company and periodically draw her attention to the meal, informing her that it is positioned on the tray's right side, because otherwise you could be guilty of unilateral neglect.

It is important that you give priority to the patient's care, and in this case you need to stay with Mrs. Biswas so that you can ensure she has looked across the entire tray to see what you have placed on it. Another reason for you to stay with this patient as she eats is to ensure her safety, because you are aware her vision is impaired. When attending to the patient, make your approach from the side of her that is not adversely affected and try your utmost to place her food within the range of vision that has not been affected. Also keep encouraging the patient to move her head in a manner to cover the entire area in front of her, otherwise she might only take notice of the items within the vision range not affected by her sight. Even when it comes to other activities, you need to guide the patient but also encourage her to do things independently, because doing things for herself promotes self-esteem.

(4)   What is one thing listed below that will not enhance the safety of your clients?

The correct answer is: (D) Always covering the client with three warm blankets at night irrespective of the weather

Safety is crucial when it comes to clients. For that reason you need to always identify the individual client before you can begin attending to him or her. You need to check the client's ID badge or bracelet and match it against your assignment sheet to ensure you are dealing with the patient you think you are. It is therefore important that clients in a nursing facility always wear their identification badges or bracelets. For further safety, CNAs are supposed to keep checking on the clients, and this is particularly important for clients who are known to have poor judgment or poor memory.

(5)    Which of the following is most likely to increase constipation?

The correct answer is: (B) Irregular bowel movements.

The term 'constipation' is used in reference to passing of stool that is hard and dry. When patients have constipation, they are bound to strain when they are having a bowel movement. Because of the discomfort, sometimes people refrain from visiting the toilet even when they feel the urge, and this worsens constipation. Other times people try to relieve themselves at odd times without necessarily having the natural urge, and this also increases the chances of developing constipation. The other options, (A), (C) and (D) serve to reduce the chances of developing constipation. Exercising a lot enhances digestive function just as consuming a diet that is high in fiber does. When the digestive system is working optimally, there is less chance of a person developing constipation. As for consuming contaminated food or water, this is more likely to cause diarrhea than constipation. Other factors that increase the risk of constipation include failure to drink sufficient fluids, certain medications, particular illnesses and aging.

(6)    What measure is most appropriate to take with a resident who has fecal incontinence?

The correct answer is: (B) Assist the resident with elimination every two or three hours after meals; give proper care to the resident's skin after elimination; use products meant for incontinence and also avoid giving the resident foods that form gas, such as beans, cucumbers and cabbage.

Fecal incontinence is one's incapacity to control how feces and gas are eliminated via the anus. People with such an issue may require bowel training, and they need to be assisted with elimination every two to three hours after meals. Products associated with incontinence are recommended because they help to keep the sheets and resident's clothing clean. It is also important to treat the resident's skin properly after elimination not only for hygiene purposes but also to ensure the skin is kept dry. Avoiding foods that are known to cause a lot of stomach gas is a good idea as well.

(7)   The doctor has issued orders that a resident who has an indwelling catheter be given bladder training. From the options listed below, choose the one that best describes the purpose of bladder training.

The correct answer is: (D) To facilitate the resident's control when he urinates.

The basic aim of bladder training is to help a person regain control of urination. Some people's urinary incontinence is actually alleviated after undergoing bladder training. The more residents have control of their urination, the more comfortable they feel. They enjoy a better quality life when incontinence ceases to be an issue. The CNA is required to help residents with bladder training only as per the direction of the nurse and the particular resident's health care plan.

(8)   There is a new CNA in your unit called Rispa and the nurse has instructed her to take a patient's rectal temperature. Which of the following is a procedure you notice Rispa is following incorrectly?

The correct answer is: (B) Telling the patient what is going to happen in the procedure and helping him lie on his right side.

Option (B) is the suitable answer because Rispa isn't handling the procedure completely correctly. The first part that involves telling the patient what is going on is appropriate, as it is important to brief the patient on what to expect of the procedure before it is done. Such explanation alleviates anxiety and fear. However, when preparing to take rectal temperature a patient should lie his or her left and not the right side. This means Rispa is trying to position the patient incorrectly. The reason this matters is that when a patient is lying on the left, it is easier and more convenient for the CNA or nurse to insert the probe as needed into the patient's anus, because it will be following the colon's position as per the anatomy of the body. Apart from option (B), all the other options contain actions that are helpful and appropriate when taking a rectal temperature.

(9)    One of the patients just admitted to the hospital unit where Mary, a CNA, is working needs his blood pressure (BP) taken on an hourly basis as per the physician's orders. It is now 15 minutes to the next BP taking and Mary has noticed the cuff provided for use is not big enough for the patient's arm; meaning if used it will be too tight. If Mary uses this cuff, the patient's BP reading is bound to _____.

The correct answer is: (B) Be above the level of the patient's actual blood pressure

Whenever the cuff used for blood pressure reading is too tight, the outcome is a BP reading that is above the actual BP the patient has. The inverse is also true—when the cuff is too loose, the BP reading is lower than the patient's actual BP. Clearly then, option (A) is incorrect. It is important that CNAs and other staff members involved use appropriately sized sphygmomanometers, or BP cuffs, whenever taking patients' blood pressure. Option (C) is incorrect as it does not spell out what inconsistency will be involved, and option (D) is outright incorrect.


(10)  Whenever you are providing oral care to a patient who is unconscious you need to be very careful, particularly in preventing fluid aspiration into the patient's lungs. Which of the following is most effective in preventing fluid aspiration?

The correct answer is: (C) Putting the patient in a position where he is lying on his side while lowering his bed.

It is expected that whenever you provide oral care to an unconscious or comatose patient, you will ensure his or her head is turned to one side. For cleaning, swab the patient's mouth progressively while also swabbing the mucous membrane using appropriate tools and supplies. As you clean out any food remnants, ensure you do not cause the patient to aspirate by inadvertently pulling food particles or fluid into his or her air passage.

Option (A) is incorrect because although you may protect the patient from getting wet by placing a towel beneath the chin, this move can't protect the patient from aspiration. Handwashing and observing hygiene is mandatory, but the question is about prevention of aspiration and therefore option (B) does not provide the solution. The actions described in option (D) about carefully cleaning the patient's mouth with swabs are good for the patient, but they do not address the issue of protection against aspiration. As such, options (A), (B) and (D) are unsuitable answers.

(11)   You are a CNA working in a nursing facility and a diabetic patient is assigned to you for care. This afternoon you are preparing to demonstrate to the patient how best to take care of his feet. Which of the following is appropriate procedure for a diabetic patient to follow?

The correct answer is: (D) Applying lotion on the feet to moisturize them and prevent dryness while avoiding the spaces between toes.

It is correct that a diabetic should have his or her feet moisturized. It is also correct that no lotion should be applied in between the toes because that raises the risk of fungal infection in those areas. There are some standard guidelines for taking care of feet, among them washing feet on a daily basis and ensuring they have been properly wiped dry especially within the spaces between the toes.

It is also recommended that toenails be trimmed whenever they have grown enough to be clipped, and they should be trimmed straight across and filed. Another recommendation is to always wear socks accompanied by shoes and avoid walking barefoot. Shoes should fit comfortably and have no rough parts inside. Another foot care guideline is avoiding exposure of feet to either heat or cold. This means wearing shoes or sandals when walking along sandy beaches and hot pavement. Diabetics should put their feet up when seated so as to enhance blood circulation to the feet. They should also wiggle their toes and move their ankles upwards and downwards twice or three times in a day. Diabetics are advised to avoid crossing their legs for long durations.


(12)   Patients with Cheyne-Stokes respiration have been known to also suffer from apnea. How do you define apnea?

The correct answer is: (C) The patient stops breathing for upwards of 15 seconds.

Sleep apnea is a breathing disorder that affects sleep, where a person's breathing is interrupted while he or she is sleeping. However, apnea in this question is in relation to a patient who has Cheyne-Stokes respiration.

Cheyne-Stokes respiration involves a pattern of abnormal breathing, where the person's breaths can be progressively deep and sometimes extra fast, and then what follows is a decline in the rate of breaths taken every moment and in due course that decline progresses to a stop in breathing; albeit temporary. This abnormal breathing pattern can repeat itself for periods ranging from 30 seconds to two minutes. Apnea as described in this question should not be confused with orthopnea, which is essentially the condition described by option (B) where the patient is unable to breathe when in the supine position. As for the condition described in option (A) where the patient has respirations that are slow and shallow and at times irregular—the correct term for that is hypoventilation.

(13)  The physician has ordered a colonoscopy for 52-year-old Amina Jones. Before ordering this procedure, the physician orders that Jones be given a enema for cleansing purposes. The position Jones should be in for this procedure is _____.

The correct answer is: (B) Sims left-lateral

When the patient is in the Sims left-lateral position, it's easy to insert the probe right into the patient's colon because of the colon's anatomical location on the left side. To be in this position, the patient's upper leg is flexed. In the meantime, the patient's lower arm is tucked behind the body. This position is also called 'semi-prone side position.'

(14)  It is time to deliver Mrs. Don's meal tray to her room. Mrs. Don is a 68-year-old resident at a nursing facility and a stroke survivor who now lives with moderate dysphagia and a few neurological deficits. Which of the following is an incorrect statement to make about a patient with dysphagia?

The correct answer is: (D) There is no reason why the patient should be assisted when eating.

The reason option (D) is the correct answer is that it is an incorrect statement regarding a patient with dysphagia. The term 'dysphagia' means difficulty in swallowing, meaning it takes a long time to get food from the mouth to the stomach. Dysphagia puts patients at high risk of aspiration, and so at no time should patients with this problem be left to eat on their own.

Option (A) is a correct statement and therefore an inappropriate answer because in this situation there is no need for the CNA to clean the patient's mouth to ensure there are no food particles that can lead to aspiration.

Option (B) is also a correct statement pertaining to a patient with dysphagia, because this position greatly reduces the risk of the patient suffering aspiration. In addition, the CNA should ensure the food being fed to the patient has consistency in its thickness. Food for a patient with dysphagia should be specially prepared for consistent ease of swallowing and is referred to as a 'dysphagia diet.'

(15)   A doctor attending a patient in a facility where you are working as a CNA asks for a pair of sterile scissors. There is one pair of scissors on a locker nearby that is still in its factory wrapping, but it is clear it has been opened and then taped closed again. What action should you take?

The correct answer is: (D) Get a new pair of sterile scissors for the doctor to use.

The reason option (D) is the correct answer is that the only way you can assume medical supplies are sterile is to check that their original seal is intact. Option (A) is incorrect because there is no room to assume tools being used on a patient are sterile; one needs to be certain. Option (B) is also incorrect because an intact seal is the confirmation you require, not another staff member's word. Also, there is no need to check the facility's manual pertaining to supplies that have been opened because some medical principles are universal.

The sterile technique stipulates that as soon as an object that was sterile when sealed is opened it is considered no longer sterile even when it has not been put to use. The reasoning behind this principle is that even if nobody touches the object, icroorganisms that are airborne are likely to begin infiltrating that object. Medical personnel and CNAs are advised to assume an object is not sterile whenever there is some doubt.

(16)   Sometimes a physician may recommend a back massage for a patient. When you are giving a back massage, what is the best position for the patient to be in?

The correct answer is: (C) the prone position.

The prone position is where the patient lies facing down, and it is the preferred position when you are giving a back massage as the patient's body directly faces you. This also allows for proper body mechanics. Option (A) is incorrect as it suggests the patient be placed in a supine position, yet in that position the patient would be facing up. This means the part of the body recommended for a massage, which is the back, will be out of your sight and reach. Option (D) is incorrect since the Fowler position does not allow for proper body mechanics when giving the patient a back massage. The Fowler position involves the patient being seated in an upright position so that the upper body and lower body are almost at a right angle.

(17) When you are giving a bed bath to a client, the recommended sequence is
_____.

The correct answer is: (A) Face first, then arms followed by chest and then the legs, back and buttocks.

The reason option (A) is the correct answer is that it follows the principle recommended when assisting a patient in bathing. The principle requires that you bathe the patient starting from the least dirty part of the body and move toward the dirtiest. The logic is that it avoids instances of microorganisms spreading from the patient's dirty areas of the body to the cleaner areas.

(18) CNAs are sometimes called upon to do some heavy lifting, and it is important that they protect themselves as they perform their duties. When trying to move a patient or heavy object from one location to another, the CNA should keep the workload as close as possible to the center of gravity in order to prevent fatigue and muscle strain.
Which of the following demonstrates the best way for a CNA to carry someone or something heavy from one point to another?

The correct answer is: (B) Ensure the person or object being carried is as close as possible to your body.

Keeping the person or the object you are trying to relocate close to your body is key. You should also avoid bending and reaching unless absolutely necessary. The patient's bed should also be raised so that it is level with your waist as much as possible.

From these principles, it is clear option (A) is incorrect as it negates the principle of being close to the work location. Option (C) is incorrect on the grounds that it negates the principle of ensuring the bed is raised to a level close to your waist. Also when you extend your arms, you end up creating a distance between you and the person or object you are carrying, and you need to have the person or object as close to your body as possible. That is the reason option (D) is incorrect.

(19) Mrs. Rodriguez has a nasogastric tube. The normal position for Mrs. Rodriguez to be in when being fed, unless it is contraindicated, is _____.

The correct answer is: (D) High Fowler's

The High Fowler's position is recommended for patients with a nasogastric tube during feeding as it improves the solution's gravitational flow and minimizes the risk of aspiration. If the solution the patient is being fed does not flow down well, there is a chance the patient could aspirate fluid into his or her lungs, which is dangerous for respiratory function.

(20) A resident in the unit you are working in has an infection that is bacterial and very virulent. Which of the following is the best precautionary measure to avoid the possible spread of the bacterial infection?

The correct answer is: (C) contact precautions.

In order to prevent the possible spread of a bacterial infection from a patient who is ill to anyone else, standard precautions should be adhered to. These include washing of hands, cleaning and disinfecting items that the patient has been in contact with and wearing personal protective equipment. Nevertheless, in this question there is no choice of standard precautions among the list of answer options, and so the most appropriate answer is contact precautions as indicated in option (C). Contact precautions include handwashing with water and soap or using a hand sanitizer as you enter the patient's room and also as you leave. You should also wear gloves and a gown while in a room with a patient and remove the glove and gown as you prepare to leave the room.

(21) Janice is an elderly patient who has just been admitted to the nursing facility and brought to the unit where you are working, and she is a first-timer at the facility. Which of the following procedures will ensure Janice's safety?

The correct answer is: (B) Ensure no furniture is in the way.

Option (B) is the best answer because for a patient who is not only elderly but also new to a facility, it is crucial that all pieces of furniture and medical equipment be kept out of the way to ensure Janice does not stumble on them. The idea is to keep common areas clear and free of clutter for patients' safety. In nursing facilities, keeping the lights on and the side rails up is always mandatory, and so these would not be changes made because of a new elderly resident. Option (C) is not at all correct because keeping every piece of equipment out of sight would not serve any purpose.

(22)  Mr. Castrol, aged 56, has chronic bronchitis. Which of the following will not enhance his respiratory function?

The correct answer is: (A) Reducing smoking.

The reason option (A) is the correct answer is that a patient with chronic bronchitis should actually quit smoking. It is not sufficient to reduce the rate of smoking as any smoking will still interfere with proper respiratory function.

The activities in option (B) contribute to enhancing respiration function because when there is deep breathing, absorption of oxygen into the bloodstream is higher and that means removal of carbon dioxide from the blood is just as high. As for increased fluid intake, it works not only by lessening dehydration but by lessening the viscosity of mucus. Patients with chronic bronchitis often have thick mucus that can be sticky, and this is one of the major reasons respiration is inhibited. Thinning of the mucus is therefore bound to improve respiratory function.

As for frequently turning a bedridden patient with chronic bronchitis, this is helpful because it reduces the chances mucus will pool within the patient's respiratory tract. Coughing can also be encouraged as an exercise to try and loosen the pooled mucus, because such an intervention also reduces chances of infection.

(23)  Georgina is giving a patient a bed path when she notices the Foley catheter is no longer taped on the anterior part of the patient's thigh. Georgina decides to correct that anomaly by obtaining some medical tape and securing the Foley catheter back in place. The rationale behind a urethral catheter's lateral anchoring, otherwise termed upward anchoring, when it applies to a male patient, is _____.

The correct answer is: (D) It helps ensure there is no pressure within the patient's penescrotal region.

The reason option (D) is the correct answer is that lateral techniques, which can also be said to be upward techniques, used in anchoring a patient's urethral catheter in a male patient serve to avoid putting pressure on the patient's penescrotal region. Securing the catheter in this manner also ensures tissue ischemia is avoided. Ischemia occurs when oxygen does not reach body cells properly because the blood reaching the tissues is restricted. If this problem persists, tissues can be damaged.

(24)  Which of the following best describes the purpose of an enema?

The correct answer is: (D) To facilitate stimulation of peristalsis.

An enema is a procedure involving injection of a liquid or gas into a patient's rectum in a bid to expel the contents within the rectum. Sometimes the procedure is used for introducing medication into the rectum or to enable X-ray imaging. When it comes to a 'cleansing enema,' it is the same procedure but this time liquid is specifically used with the aim of ensuring proper stimulation of the rectum to enable bowel movement. Often the liquid injected into the patient's rectum is pre-packaged, containing different ingredients that include salt and soap.

There are some enemas described as 'oil-retention enemas' which serve as lubricants to a patient's colon and rectum, softening feces. If the question had been about these kinds of enemas, option (C) would have been correct. As for the attempt to relieve the patient of gaseous distension and flatus, a carminative enema is required. This means option (A) would have been correct if the question had been specifically about carminative enemas.

(25)  Irene is a CNA who has been working at a long-term nursing home for two years. At the beginning of her third year at the facility, a 70-year-old resident is assigned to her. As a CNA, Irene is expected to give the patient bed baths. Every time Irene gives the patient a bed bath, the first action she should take is _____.

The correct answer is: (D) To let the patient know she is about to receive a bed bath and explain the reason

While an action such as giving a bed bath may appear like a routine procedure, it is important for the CNA to alert the patient and to explain the reason for it. This makes the patient feel you have respect for him or her and want to preserve his or her dignity. It also serves to prevent anxiety on the part of the patient.

(26) Patients on a clear liquid diet should not consume _____.

The correct answer is: (C) ice cream.

The reason option (C) is the correct answer is that one of its ingredients is milk, which is not a clear liquid.

Besides gelatin, broth and popsicles, other foods that are considered clear liquids include plain water, carbonated water, flavored water, apple juice, juice from white grapes and several other fruit juices as long as they do not contain pulp. Punch, lemonade and other beverages with fruit flavors are acceptable as clear liquids, as is soda.

(27) Michelle is a 26-year-old office clerk who has been put under observation to determine whether she has an eating disorder. Michelle must be weighed on a daily basis. In order to ensure the daily weighing is accurate, a CNA should not _____.

The correct answer is: (B) Take Michelle's weight at varying times every day.

The reason option (B) is the correct answer is that it contradicts what should be done. It is important to be consistent with the timing of weight measurement when it is being done under physicians' orders. That means the intervals in between weigh-ins should be equal.

(28) Which of the following should a CNA not do when taking a radial pulse?

The correct answer is: (B) Use the thumb to palpate the artery

The reason option (B) is the correct answer is because it represents something that the CNA should avoid. Using the thumb to take a pulse rate is a mistake because the thumb has a high pulse of its own, which means the CNA might end up measuring her own pulse rate as opposed to the patient's.

The correct procedure for checking pulse when you want to do it from the wrist is placing two fingers in between bone and tendon right over the patient's radial artery. The radial artery is the one along the side of the wrist where the thumb is. After feeling the pulse, you can then begin counting the number of times you feel the beats for a period of 15 seconds. Once you get this number, multiplying it by four will give you the pulse rate in a minute.

(29) In some unfortunate instances, patients develop pressure ulcers. Signs that mark the initial stage of these ulcers include _____.

The correct answer is: (A) Skin that is still intact but erythematic and non-blanchable

Erythematic means skin has developed redness owing to capillary congestion and dilation, which sometimes signifies the presence of inflammation or infection. Skin is said to be blanchable when blanches can be seen after exerting pressure, meaning color soon reappears after pressure exertion ceases. The term 'necrosis' is used in reference to cases where all or most cells that make up an organ die or where tissue dies as a result of illness, injury or absence of blood supply.


(30) The symptoms of hyperglycemia include _____.

The correct answer is: (C) Feeling thirsty, losing weight and urinating frequently

Hyperglycemia is a condition where a patient's level of glucose in the blood is higher than normal. This condition is linked to diabetes mellitus. In addition to feeling thirsty, losing weight and urinating frequently, other symptoms of hyperglycemia include feeling weak and drowsy, being hungry often and having a mouth that is very dry, as well having leg cramps and a flushed face. Other symptoms include breath odor that is sweet; respirations that are slow, labored and deep; a weak and rapid pulse; low blood pressure; dry skin; blurred vision; nausea accompanied by vomiting; convulsions and coma.

(31)  Osteoarthritis can confine a patient to bed for long periods. As CNAs care for patients who remain on bed rest for prolonged durations, they should _____.

The correct answer is: (C) Keep turning the patient every two hours while encouraging the patient to cough and take deep breaths.

It is a basic necessity to keep turning a patient who is bedridden every two hours because that helps prevent pressure ulcers from developing. The patient also needs to be fed proper nutrition and to be encouraged to take coughs and deep breaths because that helps to prevent other medical complications, including pneumonia. Option (A) is incorrect because even as massages can be helpful in reducing a patient's physical pain, there is no need to keep the patient very still. As for option (B), the reason it is incorrect is that it suggests only passive ROM is acceptable, yet a bedridden patient benefits from both active ROM just as well as from the passive. All these exercises contribute to maintaining the integrity of the patient's skin and prevent contractures. The reason option (D) is incorrect is that although it has good suggestions about the patient coughing and taking deep breaths, it also has an error in that it advises limiting the patient's intake of fluids. A patient needs adequate fluid intake in order to avert dehydration.


(32)  Juma, a patient who was brought to the hospital three days ago, has just undergone surgery to repair his hip. It is therefore important to position Juma's legs and hips appropriately. The most suitable position for Juma is _____.

The correct answer is: (C) abduction.

Abduction is the distancing of the limb from the patient's body midline. Once a patient has undergone hip repair surgery, the best position to be put in is abduction, as it enables a prosthesis to remain in its correct position. The CNA can also make use of an abduction pillow for the sake of holding the patient's hip in a specific position as it heals, or alternatively, a splinter, which provides stabilization for the hip abduction. Sometimes use of a pillow or a splinter becomes necessary when the hip has moved out of the joint, or when the patient has had a hip fracture. It is important to note that the patient's position can be adjusted, for example, to supine or lying on the side, but whatever position the patient's body is in, abduction must be maintained.

(33) Mrs. Simpson's left arm is paralyzed and she has been in the hospital for two and a half months due to problems feeding herself. Not surprisingly, she has been relying on the CNA to help her eat. Which of the following is an incorrect statement about assisting patients with eating?

The correct answer is: (D) Use a fork when feeding the patient.

The reason option (D) is the correct answer is that it is the statement with the wrong information. It is recommended that patients be fed using spoons and not forks because forks can more easily cause injury than spoons.

It is also recommended that the spoon being used only be one-third filled with food. The other options cannot be picked as correct answers because they contain correct information. For option (A), it is true that you should serve the patient's food in the order she prefers, as this is not only considerate on your part but it also means you are giving the patient an opportunity to eat what she has an appetite for so she might eat more. Option (B) is about praying before the meal, something that is common for many people. It is courteous to ask the patient if she would like to pray so that if she does you can give her the opportunity to do so. Option (C) suggests engaging the patient in conversation which is totally appropriate. Since mealtime provides an opportunity to interact socially, it is a good idea for the CNA to engage the patient in pleasant conversation as long as care is taken not to interfere with the patient's chewing and swallowing.

(34) Mr. Wong is a 64-year-old man who only recently emigrated from Singapore. Today he appears extraordinarily agitated. As the CNA assigned to Mr. Wong, which of the following is a good activity for you to suggest Mr. Wong partake in?

The correct answer is: (C) Taking a walk daily.

As the CNA taking care of Mr. Wong, you should anticipate instruction from the nurse to take Mr. Wong for a daily walk. Walks will help distract Mr. Wong from his feelings of hostility and will calm him down.

When you accompany the patient on his walks, even when he is not incapacitated, he can see your concern and will believe that you have a genuine interest to his welfare. So walking not only keeps negative thoughts out of Mr. Wong's mind, but it also helps him to open up to you about his thoughts and feelings and concerns. This makes him less agitated. The activities suggested in the other answer options are likely to aggravate Mr. Wong's condition, making him even more agitated.

(35) The problem of stereotyping when caring for patients is that it could end up _____.

The correct answer is: (D) Causing an erroneous medical diagnosis.

Stereotyping alludes to the generalizations made about people just because they share some things in common as a community. For example, there are stereotypes regarding race or ethnic groups, followers of particular religions and so on. It is therefore important to acquire sufficient knowledge about an illness and various health practices so that caregiving can be delivered safely and effectively.

Options (A), (B) and (C) are incorrect for various reasons, one of them being that stereotyping will jeopardize cooperation with patients and family members, not enhance it. As for frustration, both the CNA and the patient can end up being affected, but there is no telling who of the two is likely to be more or less frustrated.

(36) When feeding patients in a long-term nursing facility, it is always good to be sensitive to cultural preferences. Therefore when a resident of Indian descent is under your care, you might expect his diet to incorporate _____.

The correct answer is: (C) Rice, roti and curry

The reason option (C) is the correct answer is that rice is a staple food in India and a good part of Asia. Roti, a type of flat bread, is very popular with people from the Indian community and many people of Indian origin are used to eating hot curry. To be clear, and referring back to the question about stereotyping, not all people from India like the same food, so make sure you ask the patient or his family what he likes eating, rather than assuming anything.

Owing to religious beliefs, beef and pork are unlikely to be incorporated in meals meant for people of Indian origin. This is because India has many Hindus and their religion does not permit them to eat beef. Also there are many Muslims among the Indian community, and their religion does not permit them to eat pork. As for tortillas and beans, these constitute an important part of the Mexican diet and not the Indian diet.

(37) Suppose you enter a patient's room and he tells you there are bugs all over his bed and he wants you to get rid of them, but you see no bugs. What is the best response?

The correct answer is: (B) I realize you're afraid and I'll keep you company although there are actually no bugs that I can see anywhere in your bed.

Option (B) provides the best answer because it is clear you are neither opposing the patient nor agreeing when there are clearly no bugs to be found. In this option, it has been acknowledged that the patient is fearful, meaning you appreciate he does need some kind of assistance even if it doesn't involve bug removal. You have offered to provide this help by keeping the patient company. In essence, you have avoided negating the patient's allegations but also have not rendered them credible. It is always advisable to refrain from arguing with a patient regarding what you deem to be hallucinations. Instead, you need to enhance the patient's feeling of safety, which you can only succeed in by first of all winning the patient's trust.

Hallucinations can be described as experiences of a sensory nature that occur without any outside stimulus, mostly occurring with the person wide awake. To the hallucinating patient, the images in the hallucination are real, and that is why you shouldn't argue with someone who says he sees something.

(38) John, a patient who is confused, is under the care of Jean, a CNA who has five years of experience. Every night at 8:30 p.m., Jean takes John to the bathroom before assisting him in getting settled in bed. The routine established by Jean for John exemplifies _____.

The correct answer is: (B) Establishing a consistent routine.

It is important to establish a routine for different tasks when taking care of a patient like John who is confused. Such tasks include going to the bathroom, bathing, having meals, exercising and watching TV. Patients who are confused are not able to recognize or appreciate time, and they often do not recognize people. In fact, there are cases where such people end up becoming incapable of performing normal daily activities on their own. For patients like these, scheduling individual tasks is good because it provides a sense of normalcy or order, saving them from possible anxiety.

(39)  In the report made at the end of the shift, the nurse informs the CNA that Mrs. Bradshaw, who is Jewish, has requested a meal that is a strictly kosher diet, and the information has already been relayed to the dietary section of the nursing facility. Which of the following meals is most appropriate for Mrs. Bradshaw?

The correct answer is: (D) Sweet and sour chicken, rice, vegetables, bowl of mixed fruits and juice

The reason option (D) is the correct answer is that it has neither pork nor pork products, and it also has no fish or products associated with animals that do not have scales or fins. People of the Jewish faith who adhere to a kosher diet do not consume pork or its products, and so the meal tray in option (B) cannot be served to Mrs. Bradshaw. As for the trays with fish or fish products, these cannot be served to Mrs. Bradshaw because the fish used have no fins or scales. A kosher diet only permits eating fish that have scales and fins, yet the fish used in options (A), which is crab, and option (C), which is shrimp, do not fulfill those requirements.

If a practicing Jew who observes a kosher diet wants to eat meat, he or she can only consume meat from animals that are cloven-hoofed and those that feed solely on vegetables and which are ritually slaughtered.

(40)  As a new CNA in a long-term nursing facility, your supervisor is taking you around for orientation. One of the residents approaches you and addresses you saying he does not belong at the facility and pleads with you to get him out. Which of the following is the best response?

The correct answer is: (A) Since I'm new and just being given an orientation, I'll come back and talk to you later.

This patient appears mentally disturbed and somewhat restless. Once you have introduced yourself to him saying you are a new staff member, you help him return to reality. Also, by promising to return to have a discussion with the patient, you are conveying that you consider him and what he has to say important, and that is reassuring for him. It also helps to alleviate anxiety.

It is important to note that such a response is not only for the sake of keeping peace with the patient and then to be ignored thereafter. It is important that such a patient be listened to and his fears and anxiety addressed without delay.

(41)  Which of the following is a component in the communications process?

The correct answer is: (C) Message and sender, feedback, receiver and the channel

The reason option (C) is the correct answer is that basic communication comprises five components: namely the person sending and the one receiving the communication, the medium through which that communication is taking place, the factors involved in the particular context, the information or message being communicated and then the feedback given. Other answer options do not provide real communication components. Like option (D), for example, what it provides are examples of non-verbal communication.

(42)  During his orientation at a new nursing facility, the nurse who is to be CNA Jason's supervisor emphasizes the need for CNAs and all staff comprising the health team to be well coordinated and communicate with one another in order to provide the best possible care to residents. Which of the following will not help enhance communication?

The correct answer is: (D) Making use of terms that have a range of meanings.

The reason option (D) is the appropriate answer is that it contains the action Jason should not take as a CNA, which is to use words that have a range of meanings. Using such words is likely to cause ambiguity or confusion in communication, and this can put a patient's health or life at risk.

It is crucial that every word used bears the same meaning in the mind of the speaker as it does in that of the listener. For effective communication, it is also advisable to use words that are familiar, especially when communicating to the patient or the patient's family members. Being brief and concise is also a basic necessity for everyone involved in providing care for residents. To succeed in this, staff need to avoid venturing into topics or issues unrelated to the idea or piece of information being relayed. In short, CNAs and other staff providing health care should strive to stay on the subject at hand. It is also important that you present your thoughts in an orderly fashion. Giving information one step at a time is very helpful. Giving facts and being specific makes communication more clear. For example, it's better to say that the patient's pulse rate was 110 rather than merely saying it was fast. The latter would leave the listener guessing and imagining different numbers for the patient's pulse rate.

(43) Communication is considered ongoing, dynamic and a multi-dimensional process. Which of communication's components is referred to as 'decoder'?

The correct answer is: (D) The receiver.

The reason option (D) is the correct answer is that the receiver of communication is the one who also decodes it to get the intended message. The referent in option (A) is not correct because the role of the referent is to motivate an individual to enter into communication with another.

Option (B), the sender, is incorrect because the role of the sender is to encode the message and deliver it. Option (C) cannot be correct because it represents the message that the receiver sends back after receiving the initial message from the sender.

(44) CNAs are not licensed nurses, and although their work is very important in the health care sector there are some tasks they are not permitted to undertake. Which of the following is not a task you should refuse to carry out?

The correct answer is: (A) A task you have always disliked.

As a CNA, it is not within your rights to refuse to carry out a task because you don't like it. All the other options have valid reasons for you to refuse carrying out the tasks. There are some tasks you can only carry out under direct supervision of a licensed nurse, and overall the tasks you carry out should only be those spelled out in the job description. Performing a task that is beyond the scope of your mandate as CNA makes you liable if a patient is harmed in any way. Another acceptable reason for choosing not to perform a task is if you don't know how to carry it out correctly and perhaps require more training. Also, if in your judgment an action has the potential to harm a patient, you should refrain. If the patient's health changes from the time you are asked to perform the task to when you go to perform it, and now it seems the task is contraindicated, you can refrain from carrying out the task. You are also free to refuse to carry out a task if it involves equipment you are not familiar with or if the directions provided are not clear. At the same time, if you deem the directions given to you to be unethical or if they contradict any policy of the facility or are outright illegal, you should refuse to follow them.

(45) Which of the following is correct about an advance directive?

The correct answer is: (B) The doctor has already assessed the wishes as stated in the document with the intention of determining what the patient wants or does not want.

An advance directive is a legal document describing the patient's wishes pertaining to his or her own health care, which are meant to guide everyone involved when the patient is no longer able to make decisions or choices.

However, advance directives are quite different from Do Not Resuscitate (DNR) orders. It is also important to note that these advance directives cannot be implemented when the person concerned is able to comprehend things and make decisions about himself or herself. Another important point to note is that there are three steps to be followed before determining an advance directive can be implemented. First, a doctor must certify that the patient no longer has the capacity to make decisions. Second, the doctor must make a diagnosis and establish a patient's prognosis. And third, the doctor must evaluate the patient's wishes as stated in the document to determine what the patient wants and does not want. Other terms used in place of 'advance directive' are 'living will,' 'medical directive' and 'advance decision.'

(46) Which of the following is correct about conferences held in a nursing facility?

The correct answer is: (D) Residents can refuse any of the suggestions the health care team makes.

There are two different kinds of conferences pertaining to resident care that OBRA provides for. One of them is the Interdisciplinary Care Planning (IDCP) conference, and the other is conferences focused on solving problems. The former is held on a regular basis with a view to developing, reviewing and updating health care plans. This conference is attended by physicians and licensed nurses as well as other members of health care teams. Residents in the nursing home and their family members can also be in attendance. The latter conferences are held only when there are specific problems affecting the care of individual residents. As such, the members of staff expected to attend are those directly involved in providing care to the respective clients in the area where the problem seems to exist. Affected residents and members of their families may also be required to be in attendance.

(47) Sometimes CNAs need to ask residents questions in a direct manner because there is some specific information they want to get. Which of the following exemplifies a direct question?

The correct answer is: (C) Are you feeling better this time?

The reason option (C) is correct is that it is a question that can only be answered by the singular words 'yes' or 'no.' There are some instances where such direct questions come in handy, like when the response is needed instantly or when the resident to whom the question is being directed has limited capacity to communicate. Option (A) cannot be the correct answer because it is not even a question. It is a statement. Options (B) and (D) cannot be correct because the answer anticipated in each of them cannot be a brief 'yes' or 'no.' They are questions whose answers are likely to come in the form of a longer explanation.

(48) Communication is very important in helping to provide care to patients, but sometimes there are hindrances or barriers to communication. Which of the following best exemplifies a barrier in communication?

The correct answer is: (D) Cultural variations between the nursing staff and the residents.

The reason option (D) is the correct answer is that when there are differences of a cultural nature between residents and the staff taking care of them, communication may be impeded, especially because either party may end up attaching the wrong meaning to statements made or to particular body language. Option (A) does not represent a communication barrier because sometimes having the CNA maintain total silence while being physically present can prove quite therapeutic for the resident. As for option (B), it is actually recommended that health care staff make use of abbreviations that have been universally accepted in the medical field. They make communication easier and faster. Option (C), which entails communication through interpreters, helps communication rather than hinders it.

(49) Agnes is a CNA at a nursing facility, and she has overheard a colleague speak of the nurse in charge of their floor being in an illicit relationship with one of the physicians. Agnes has decided to give this information to her supervising nurse. Which of the following is the best description of the situation?

The correct answer is: (A) Agnes has opted to participate in gossip and this is unprofessional behavior

Discussing other people's private affairs is gossip. It constitutes unprofessional behavior and can end up hurting other people. Refrain from discussing patients or residents, people's families or visitors, co-workers or your employer in any social setting. If people are gossiping, leave the room. It is also advisable to refrain from repeating any questionable statements which may or may not be true.


(50) Sometimes there may be a need to do a background check on a newly recruited CNA. The best authority to provide information of this nature is _____.

The correct answer is: (C) the Nursing Assistant Registry.

This registry has all relevant information pertaining to CNAs who have been trained and passed the relevant CNA exam. The registry contains CNAs' full names, last recorded home address, birth date and registration number and expiration date. Other relevant information the registry can provide includes former employers, the date a CNA was hired and the date that employment came to an end, the date the CNA exam was passed and any negative information pertaining to abuse, neglect and the like. Such information is not provided by the National Council for State Boards of Nursing (NCSBN) or the 1987 OBRA. All the relevant information regarding CNAs remains in the Nursing Assistant Registry for a minimum period of five years.


(51) CNAs and other health care providers are expected to show empathy for their clients as they take care of them. Which of the following demonstrates empathy on the part of a CNA?

The correct answer is: (B) Putting yourself in other people's shoes. Option (B) is the correct answer. When you empathize, you imagine the feelings the other person is experiencing, but you don't pity the person. Option (A) involves caring, rather than empathy, because when you care for someone you tend to put the needs of that person before your own. As for option (C) which involves doing something extra for another person, it only shows you respect that person. Option (D) involves sharing of feelings with the resident you are taking care of, and this is not empathy. It's discouraged as you want to maintain a professional relationship with residents, rather than a friendship.

(52) The most suitable time to make use of a soft Toothette is _____.

The correct answer is: (B) An unconscious client requires oral care.

The reason option (B) is the correct answer is that when dealing with a resident who is unconscious, you cannot risk using toothpaste and you cannot be sure the resident will be safe if you use any fluids. As such, Toothettes come in handy. All other options provided are incorrect.

Toothettes are oral swabs used in maintaining the teeth and gums healthy. They are used to gently remove debris from the mouth, cleaning in between individual teeth and serving as stimulants to oral tissues. Many long-term nursing facilities have Toothettes for use on patients who are very ill or weak. Sometimes Toothettes are referred to as oral swabs or sponge swabs, foam swabs or mouth swabs.

(53) There is a resident in your unit who had a stroke a few weeks ago but is now recovering. His entire left side is very weak, and now you have been requested to assist the resident to put on a warm sweater. You should provide assistance to the resident from _____.

The correct answer is: (B) The left-hand side of the resident.

The reason you need to be on the patient's left side while helping him dress is that it's the weakest side because of his stroke and therefore requires the most support. At the same time, assisting from that side helps the resident maintain his balance. All the other options cannot be considered the best.

(54) You are the CNA in charge of a resident who has Alzheimer's, and this particular day there have been very many visitors in his room who have stayed for several hours. Since it is now time for the resident to bathe, the most suitable action for you to take is

_____.

The correct answer is: (A) Ask the visitors to leave the room until the resident has completed his bath.

The reason option (A) is the most suitable answer is that the presence of the visitors for several hours in the resident's room has inhibited ADLs, and since as a CNA you are allowed to take charge where the welfare of your resident is concerned, you can confidently ask the visitors to step out of the room to give you a chance to attend to the resident.

Option (B) is not correct because bathing is an ADL, and all efforts should be made to ensure ADLs are fulfilled on a daily basis. After all, the visitors can always wait in another section of the facility as you bathe the resident. The reason option (C) is incorrect is that you need not escalate the issue of visitors to the nurse in charge as it is within your mandate to clear the room for the sake of providing care to the resident. As for option (D), it is inappropriate to ask the resident the best time for you to return as he is not in a position to make reasonable decisions regarding timing due to his Alzheimer's.

(55) There is a resident at the nursing facility who has been put on the DASH diet. The resident is eating less now and appears not to like her food. As the CNA caring for this patient, what is the best step for you to take?

The correct answer is: (D) See if the doctor has prescribed any dietary supplements and if so, make sure the resident takes them.

Among the answer choices provided, the best option is to give the resident the dietary supplements already prescribed. Option (A) is incorrect not because involving the facility nutritionist is a bad move, but because it is not for the CNA to make that call. A nurse or physician should make that decision. Also, while it may not be against the facility's policies to have residents be brought food from outside, and while the family may be willing to bring their relative her favorite food, there is no guarantee the food will match the DASH diet. This means the food might interfere with the health care recommended for the resident. That makes option (B) unsuitable. Option (C) is also not suitable because you are unlikely to succeed in getting the patient to eat bigger portions of food she does not like.

(56) Jason is required to report for physical therapy every day after breakfast, but it has become a habit for him to get there late because he feeds himself and eats his breakfast slowly. What is the correct action to take in this situation?

The correct answer is: (D) Ensure Jason is served breakfast earlier in the day.

The reason option (D) is the most appropriate answer is that by providing breakfast earlier Jason will still eat well and enjoy his meal while retaining his independence, which is something to be encouraged. The reason options (A) and (C) are unsuitable is that your actions would actually be approaching neglect. In (A) Jason would probably be going to physical therapy while hungry, and in (C) it would appear like taunting someone whose slow speed is not his fault but the result of his health status. Feeding Jason as option (B) suggests might ensure he eats adequately, but it would make him dependent while he still has the ability to care for himself in this respect.


(57) Which of the following is not a typical eating challenge that residents face?

The correct answer is: (D) Forgetting when mealtime is.

The reason option (D) is the correct answer is that it should be routine at the nursing facility for residents to be reminded when mealtime is. In fact, it is incumbent upon the nursing facility to ensure the residents who cannot feed themselves have CNAs to feed them or to provide necessary assistance. Moreover, the facility is expected to provide meals in a timely manner even to residents who need to be fed intravenously. So this option cannot be termed a feeding challenge because it is an activity that residents and management anticipate every time it is time for residents to have their meals.
The other options—(A), (B) and (C)—are real mealtime challenges. A resident's inability to manipulate utensils is a real challenge as it inhibits his or her independence, and decreased capacity to recognize either hunger or thirst is a big challenge because the resident might end up either overeating or undereating. Certainly problems that inhibit residents' ability to chew or swallow qualify as mealtime challenges.

(58) Bathing residents who are weak or bedridden is one of the tasks performed by CNAs. Nevertheless, there is one important aspect associated with a resident's bathing needs that caregivers often overlook or forget, and that is_____.

The correct answer is: (B) The frequency with which people bathe varies from culture to culture.

The reason option (B) is the most suitable answer is that rarely do caregivers factor in cultural practices when preparing a resident's bathing schedule. Yet the frequency with which people normally take a bath may vary from one culture to another. In short, there is a need for caregivers to seek the opinion of the residents and assess how reasonable their usual pattern of bathing would be, and then see how best to tailor the bathing schedules of respective residents.
The other options—(A), (C) and (D)—are part of standard procedures expected to be followed every time a resident is being given a bath. So they cannot be part of the usually forgotten aspects of bathing.

(59) Although there are some standard procedures followed when providing health care to residents, there are also procedures that CNAs are expected to follow because of stipulations in a particular facility. From the procedures included in the four options below, identify the one a CNA would follow because of rules at the nursing facility.

The correct answer is: (A) toenail-cutting policy.

The reason option (A) is the best answer is that there are some nursing facilities that only permit doctors and licensed nurses to trim residents' toenails.
As for options (B), (C) and (D), those are standard procedures that CNAs are expected to perform as part of their duties, just as they are expected to avoid cutting the nails too near the flesh and to cut straight across the nail.

(60)  Many residents receiving care in long-term nursing facilities have dentures. Which of the following is a false statement about denture care?

The correct answer is: (D) Taking care of dentures is the responsibility of the residents themselves, and for that reason there is no chance of charging the nursing facility with negligence if a resident's dentures are ever damaged.

Option (D) is the preferred answer as it contains the false statement. The true position is that the facility ought to take responsibility for the welfare of the residents as well as their dentures since residents are under nursing care because they are incapacitated in one way or another. In short, it would not be reasonable to expect individual residents to always take care of their dentures all on their own. As for the other options, they are actually true as far as dentures are concerned. For example, dentures are most slippery when wet. It is also a fact that dentures are expensive and yet fragile. Using cool water to store dentures within when they are not in use is standard procedure. As such, none of these three options qualifies to be chosen as the answer for this question.

CPSIA information can be obtained
at www.ICGtesting.com
Printed in the USA
LVHW061411091020
668426LV00022B/847

9 781989 726006